Overview Ma

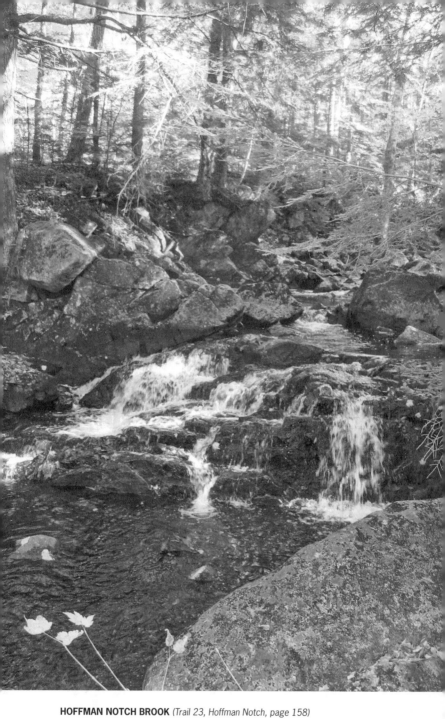

HOFFMAN NOTCH BROOK *(Trail 23, Hoffman Notch, page 158)*

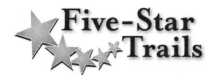

Five-Star Trails

Adirondacks

YOUR GUIDE TO 46 SPECTACULAR HIKES

TIM STARMER

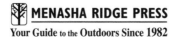

MENASHA RIDGE PRESS
Your Guide to the Outdoors Since 1982

Five-Star Trails: Adirondacks: Your Guide to 46 Spectacular Hikes

Copyright © 2017 by Tim Starmer
All rights reserved
Published by Menasha Ridge Press
Printed in the United States of America
Distributed by Publishers Group West
Second edition, second printing 2022

Cover design: Scott McGrew
Text design: Annie Long
Cartography and elevation profiles: Scott McGrew, Thomas Hertzel, and Tim Starmer
Cover and interior photos: Tim Starmer

Library of Congress Cataloging-in-Publication Data
Names: Starmer, Timothy, 1975- author.
Title: Five-star trails, Adirondacks : 40 spectacular hikes in upstate New York / Tim Starmer.
Description: Second edition. | Birmingham, Alabama : Menasha Ridge Press, 2017.
Identifiers: LCCN 2016053971 | ISBN 9781634040525 (paperback)
Subjects: LCSH: Hiking—New York (State)—Adirondack Mountains—Guidebooks. | Trails—
    New York (State)—Adirondack Mountains—Guidebooks. | Adirondack Mountains (N.Y.)—
    Guidebooks. | BISAC: TRAVEL / United States / Northeast / New England (CT, MA, ME,
    NH, RI, VT). | SPORTS & RECREATION / Hiking. | HEALTH & FITNESS / Healthy Living.
Classification: LCC GV199.42.N652 A34735 2017 | DDC 796.51097475—dc23
LC record available at https://lccn.loc.gov/2016053971

ISBN: 978-1-63404-052-5; eISBN: 978-1-63404-053-2

MENASHA RIDGE PRESS
An imprint of AdventureKEEN
2204 First Ave. S, Ste. 102
Birmingham, Alabama 35233
800-678-7006, fax 877-374-9016

Visit menasharidge.com for a complete listing of our books and for ordering information.
Contact us at our website, at facebook.com/menasharidge, or at twitter.com/menasharidge with
questions or comments. To find out more about who we are and what we're doing, visit blog
.menasharidge.com.

Contents

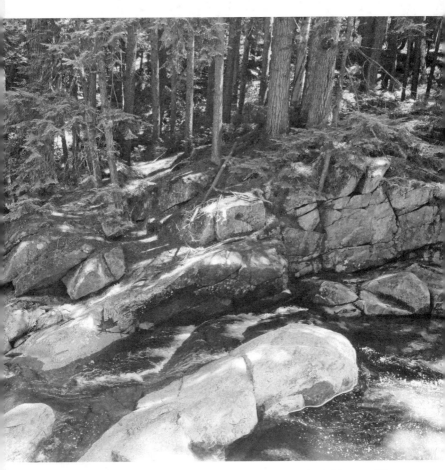

TOP OF THE FIRST FALLS ALONG TENANT CREEK *(Trail 5, Tenant Creek Falls, page 50)*

Dedication

This book is dedicated to my parents, who first inspired in me a love of the great outdoors and helped in innumerable ways in completing this book.

Acknowledgments

FIRST AND FOREMOST, I would like to thank everyone who braved the trails with me and endured my repetitious mumblings into my voice recorder. Your company was appreciated and helpful.

Second, I must acknowledge all the work that my parents contributed to this project, from editing my rough drafts to retyping hikes I lost when my computer crashed to loaning me a car when my truck broke down, sadly more than once.

Finally, I would like to acknowledge the tireless efforts of all the trail crews who maintain the thousands of miles of trails in the Adirondacks. Your work is greatly admired and appreciated.

—T. S.

Preface

WORKING ON THIS BOOK was definitely an experience to remember. I lost two hard drives; had to rewrite a handful of hikes from memory; fried a camera, a voice recorder, and a GPS unit; sprained my ankle; was nearly blown off a mountaintop; and was stranded in the middle of the Adirondacks when my truck broke down and AAA redefined 24/7 service as weekdays only during business hours. It was memorable and—quite simply—great. Planning and replanning hikes, followed by days in the woods, is more than most hikers can ask for; to do so in the Adirondacks is definitely more than most get.

For those who don't know, the Adirondack Park is huge. The park's boundaries encompass 9,375 square miles, which is larger than each of the states of Rhode Island, Delaware, Connecticut, New Jersey, and New Hampshire. It is only 240 square miles smaller than Vermont. Compared to national parks, the Adirondack Park is larger than Grand Canyon, Yellowstone, Yosemite, Great Smoky Mountains, and Big Bend National Parks combined. In fact, its boundaries, also known as the blue line, encompass more acreage than any of the national parks in the Lower 48 states. Not all of the land within the blue line is owned or managed by the state. Towns, villages, and two entire counties, as well as vast tracts of privately held land, lie within its boundaries. However, don't let the land classification fool you—the park is truly a vast wilderness. Of the 6.1 million acres, almost 45%, or 2.6 million acres, is owned by the state, though donations and purchases continue to expand the state-owned land. Of the remaining land, less than 1% is municipal property and about 6% is classified as low-level residential, which is almost equivalent to the amount of acreage of water within the park. The remaining land is either rural or privately owned forests.

No matter how you frame it, the park is a huge wilderness, and you sense it almost immediately after passing the blue line. As you drive toward any of the hundreds of trailheads, you can feel the forest encroaching on the fields and houses along the roads. You know that the boundary between civilization and a sprawling wilderness is just beyond the treeline. Soon the forests have overrun manicured lawns, and fields give way to staggering boulders and craggy cliffs that loom close to the roadside. You sense that at any point, you could stop your car, step out into the woods, and within feet completely leave civilization behind. All the while, should you choose to stop at a diner for lunch in between hikes, forget camera batteries, need to refuel, or need replacement gear, there is typically a spot to resupply within a half hour of a trailhead. This is the charm of the Adirondacks: A vast wilderness, in which you can spend days in solitude, is at your fingertips, and yet civilization is still close at hand. For many beginning hikers, this is a great comfort, while experienced hikers can revel in the idea of a warm meal or cold drink at the end of a journey.

My goal in writing this book was to cater to both beginning and experienced hikers by providing easy and challenging hikes in all corners of the park. I could have easily found 40-plus hikes in any single region, and all would have been rewarding. Some of the hikes will be familiar, others less known, but all are rewarding examples of the many facets of the Adirondack Park and its thousands of miles of trails.

—*Tim Starmer*

Recommended Hikes

Best for Solitude

Best for Waterfalls

Best for Lakes and Ponds

Best for Mountains

Easiest Hikes

Most Challenging Hikes

Best for Fall Colors

Best for Wheelchair Accessibility (portions)

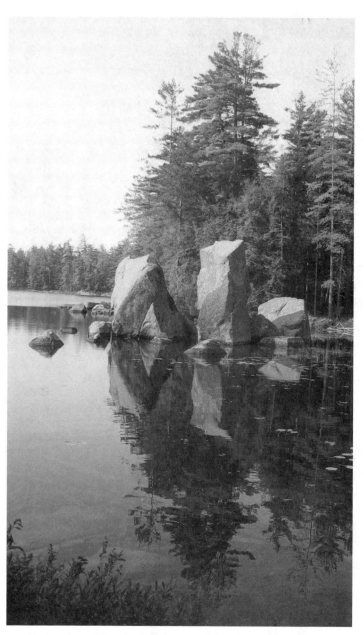

SPLIT ROCK BAY ON PHARAOH LAKE *(Trail 29, Pharaoh Lake, page 197)*

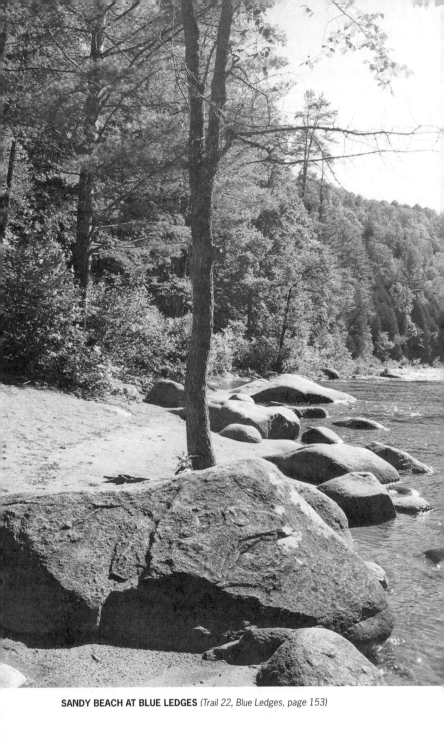

SANDY BEACH AT BLUE LEDGES (Trail 22, Blue Ledges, page 153)

Introduction

About This Book

AN ESTIMATED 6 MILLION–10 MILLION TOURISTS visit Adirondack Park every year. With 3,000 lakes, 30,000 miles of rivers and streams, 2,000 miles of hiking trails, and more than 100 mountains, it is no surprise. *Unique* is barely adequate to describe the character of the Adirondacks. It stands out as the largest park in the Lower 48 states; however, unlike its rivals, it's managed solely by the state. It has the only mountains in the Northeast that are not geologically Appalachian. The mountains, though geologically new, are from old rock. Ecologically, the park lies on the transition of the boreal forests of the north and deciduous hardwood forests of the south. The Adirondack region was also at the forefront of conservation when, in 1894, the Forever Wild character of the forest preserve was added to the state constitution, making it the first preserve with constitutional protection.

New mountains from old rock seem a contradiction, but this is what makes the Adirondack Mountains distinct from their Appalachian neighbors along the East Coast. Unlike the Appalachian Mountains, which were formed by plate tectonics, the Adirondack Mountains were formed by uplift. Indeed, the Adirondacks are still rising. Granted, the rate is only about 3 millimeters per year, but this rate is faster than the rate of erosion, so the mountains are creeping ever upward. So the next time someone comments that life was tougher in his day, you can quip that at least his mountains were shorter.

The protruding old rock was formed when the Adirondacks were part of a giant inland sea. Over millennia, miles of sediment were deposited and later transformed by high pressure and heat into metamorphosed rock. The deposits and formation took place 1 billion years ago, and the metamorphosed rock lay miles beneath the surface until erosion removed enough material for a 160-mile-wide bulge to begin swelling above the surrounding landscape about

5 million years ago. Further stages of uplift, erosion, and the scouring of the landscape by great ice sheets have exposed the metamorphosed rock and caused the uplift to increase. These powerful forces of uplift, erosion, and scouring transformed the region into the rugged wilderness we see today.

American Indians did not settle in the Adirondacks, but rather used them mostly as hunting grounds. As Europeans began to explore and settle the continent, they stayed on the fringes of the wilderness, mostly along the shores of Lake George and Lake Champlain. These lakes formed a major strategic territory for mastery of the continent. The Iroquois and Algonquin often fought over the water route long before the pitched battles of the French and Indian War. During this war, the French controlled Fort Carillon, later named Fort Ticonderoga, on the northern shore of Lake Champlain, while the English controlled Fort William Henry on the south end. James Fenimore Cooper's novel *The Last of the Mohicans* depicts one of the major events in this contest over the water route: the surrender of Fort William Henry followed by a massacre of the retreating English troops on their way to Fort Edward. The magnitude of the massacre has been estimated from dozens to thousands, though it is generally agreed that Cooper's depiction is exaggerated. Later epic battles were fought during this war and then again during the American Revolution. However, during all this time, the interior of the Adirondack wilderness was rarely broached.

Settlement in the region did not begin in earnest until the 1800s, when the Industrial Revolution's growing demand for natural resources turned its eyes on the vast stands of timber and newly discovered veins of iron ore. Great wealth was created during the Gilded Age, and consequently, the Adirondacks became a popular vacation area with great camps and resorts. At the same time, conservation and a love of the outdoors were taking hold of the public, and the devastation of the Adirondack forests became a growing concern among these newly arrived vacationers. In 1885 the state created the Adirondack Forest Preserve, which directed that "the lands now or hereafter constituting the Forest Preserve shall be forever kept as wild forest lands." Later in 1892 the state established the Adirondack State Park and drew the infamous blue line to encompass the Adirondack Forest Preserve, as well as millions of acres of private land. Despite these protections, the forest preserve law was still violated; in 1894 the "forever wild" clause was added to the state constitution of New York. Tourism continued to thrive in the region and saw increases after World War I and World War II. Second homes within the park became a growing concern, and in 1971 the Adirondack Park Agency was created to develop and oversee land-use plans with consideration of the "forever wild" clause.

Today the park still maintains a delicate balance between the interests of private landholders and the public lands owned by the state. To say that tourism is a mainstay of the region is an understatement. There are 130,000 people living year-round in the 9,375 square miles encompassed by the blue line, with an estimated 200,000 seasonal residents and anywhere from 6 million to 10 million tourists. So odds are that if you ask someone for directions, the person won't be from around there. Tourism is year-round, with winter attracting snowmobilers, skiers, and snowshoers in as many numbers as summer's vacationers and fall's hunters. About the only downtime is in early spring during the mud season.

The hikes within this book are meant to provide a wide range of experiences over the vast area of the park. For decades the park has informally been divided into regions in various ways. The Department of Environmental Conservation (DEC) has regions that sprawl across the blue line; counties divide the park but also cross the line; and varying tourist centers divide the region based on proximity to major lakes or towns.

Most people adhere to the six regions originally devised by the Adirondack Mountain Club (ADK) in its earlier versions of the Forest Preserve series of guidebooks. I have similarly divided the region because it proves useful for hikers seeking nearby trails or additional maps and is generally understood by most hikers as the way the park is divided. Though regions often overlap, some distinctions between the regions help to describe the area to be explored.

Southern Region

The southern foothills are not known for their mountains, so it may seem odd that the two mountains featured here are actually some of the steepest hikes. They are not as tall as those in the High Peaks, but their straight-up ascents make them reasonably challenging, yet well within the novice hiker's range. Similar to the west-central and central regions, the terrain here is mostly level, and lakes and other bodies of water are the primary focus of trails. Several unmarked trails are also featured in this region but are easy to follow with a little navigational experience.

West-Central Region

Along the western border of the park are the foothills that lead to the Adirondack Mountains. Few mountains are in this area; most trails follow the shores of lakes and rivers and feature generally flat terrain. The few mountain trails in this area are well liked, so expect lots of company. Indeed, the region, especially around the towns of Old Forge and Inlet, is extremely popular with tourists. Many of the great camps were built here, and it serves as a staging point for longer expeditions into the Adirondacks. Several excellent campgrounds, outdoors stores, and outfitters are in the area, making it a good point to resupply or pick up forgotten items as you head deeper into the park. It does not take long to leave the vestiges of civilization behind here, so the purist should not shun this region simply because it is well known.

Central Region

As might be expected, the central region lies in the center of many of the other Adirondack regions; consequently, many of its trailheads lie literally across the street from a trail in another region. Many of the trails described in this region are unmarked and considered bushwhacks but generally are well trodden. Additionally, these trails follow the course of streams, so navigating them should be relatively easy. The area is essentially bound by NY 28 to the north and NY 8 to the south. Several mountains are in this region, though most are easy to climb. An abundance of waterfalls in this region makes it an excellent area for exploring waterscapes. Many of the campgrounds in the area provide solitude and scenery, making them excellent staging areas for exploring all the regions in the park.

Eastern Region

Hikes in this region focus on the shores of Lake George and feature spectacular vistas from the mountains that surround the beautiful lake. The southern tip of Lake George is full of tourist trappings and won't be high on the list for most devoted hikers. However, it does provide a good staging area, the opportunity to reconnect with civilization, and quick access to the excellent wilderness areas nearby. Pharaoh Lake and Mountain are featured in the book but cover just a small portion of the vast Pharaoh Lake Wilderness Area.

Northern Region

The northern region looks and feels like a giant river basin. The mostly level terrain is dotted with innumerable ponds, lakes, and marshes, which are all bisected by a network of streams and winding rivers. The Floodwood and High Falls loops described in this guide typify the region and are fascinating areas to explore. Not as built-up or commercial as other areas in the park, the northern region is definitely the most remote and probably the hardest area in which to resupply. Cranberry Lake, Tupper Lake, and Saranac are the largest developed areas, but you'll pass through them quickly. Hikes here are generally more secluded; however, as is the case in most regions, the peaks attract the most hikers.

High Peaks Region

Rugged and wild, the High Peaks typify the Adirondacks. Hikers who put off venturing into the High Peaks region for decades often never return to their earlier stomping grounds once they get a taste of the High Peaks. Generally, trails here are steeper, cliffs and waterfalls are taller, and the sheer quantity of peaks in this region changes your view of what rugged looks and feels like. This book offers just a sampling of the adventures that lie in the High Peaks and leans toward the beginner level for the region. However, beginner High Peaks trails are typically more difficult than more advanced trails in other regions.

How to Use This Guidebook
Overview Map, Map Key, and Map Legend

The overview map on the inside front cover depicts the location of the primary trailhead for all of the hikes described in this book. Each hike's number appears on the overview map, on the map key facing the overview map, and in the table of contents. A hike's full profile is easy to locate as you flip through the book—just watch for the hike number at the top of each page. A map legend that details the symbols found on trail maps appears on the inside back cover.

Trail Maps

Each hike contains a detailed map that shows the trailhead, the complete route, significant features, facilities, and topographic landmarks such as creeks, overlooks, and peaks. I gathered map data by carrying a GPS unit (Garmin eTrex) while hiking each route, and then sent that data to the publisher's expert cartographers. However, your GPS is not really a substitute for sound, sensible navigation that takes into account the conditions you observe while hiking.

Further, despite the high quality of the maps in this guidebook, the publisher and author strongly recommend that you always carry an additional map, such as the ones noted in each entry opener's listing for "Maps."

Elevation Profiles

The elevation profile represents the rises and falls of the trail as viewed from the side, over the complete distance (in miles) of that trail. On the diagram's vertical axis, or height scale, the number of feet indicated between each tick mark lets you visualize the climb. To avoid making flat hikes look steep and steep hikes appear flat, varying height scales provide an accurate image of each hike's climbing challenge. For example, one hike's scale might rise to 800 feet, while another goes to 6,000 feet.

Also, each entry's opener will list the elevation at the hike trailhead, and it will list the elevation peak.

The Hike Profile

Each hike profile opens with the hike's star ratings, GPS trailhead coordinates, and other key at-a-glance information—from the trail's distance and configuration to contacts for local information. Each profile also includes a map (see "Trail Maps," page 6). The main text for each profile includes three sections: "Overview," "Route Details," and "Directions" (for driving to the trailhead area).

Flip through the book, read the "Overview" summaries, and choose the hikes that appeal to you. A list of recommended hikes (see pages xi–xii) will also help you choose a hike to fit your mood and group.

Star Ratings

The hikes in *Five-Star Trails: Adirondacks* were carefully chosen to give the hiker an overall five-star experience and represent the diversity of trails found in the region. Each hike was assigned a one- to five-star rating in each of the following categories: scenery, trail condition, suitability for children, level of difficulty, and degree of solitude. While one hike may merit five stars for its stunning scenery, that same trail may rank as a two-star trail for children. Similarly, another hike might receive two stars for difficulty but earn five stars for solitude. It's rare that any trail receives five stars in all five categories; nevertheless, each trail offers excellence in at least one category, if not others. Here's how the star ratings for each of the five categories break down:

FOR SCENERY:

★★★★★	Unique, picturesque panoramas
★★★★	Diverse vistas
★★★	Pleasant views
★★	Unchanging landscape
★	Not selected for scenery

FOR TRAIL CONDITION:

★★★★★	Consistently well maintained
★★★★	Stable, with no surprises
★★★	Average terrain to negotiate
★★	Inconsistent, with good and poor areas
★	Rocky, overgrown, or often muddy

FOR CHILDREN:

★★★★★	Excellent choice for introducing young kids to hiking
★★★★	Fun for anyone past the toddler stage with some hiking experience
★★★	Good for young hikers with proven stamina
★★	Not enjoyable for children
★	Not advisable for children

FOR DIFFICULTY:

★★★★★	Grueling
★★★★	Strenuous
★★★	Moderate (won't beat you up—but you'll know you've been hiking)
★★	Easy with patches of moderate
★	Good for a relaxing stroll

FOR SOLITUDE:

★★★★★	Positively tranquil
★★★★	Spurts of isolation
★★★	Moderately secluded
★★	Crowded on weekends and holidays
★	Steady stream of individuals and/or groups

GPS Trailhead Coordinates

As noted in "Trail Maps" on page 6, I used a handheld GPS unit to obtain geographic data and sent the information to the publisher's cartographers. In the opener for each hike profile, the coordinates—the intersection of the latitude (north) and longitude (west)—will orient you from the trailhead. In some cases, you can drive within viewing distance of a trailhead. Other hiking routes require a short walk to the trailhead from a parking area.

You will also note that this guidebook uses the degree–decimal minute format for presenting the latitude and longitude GPS coordinates. The latitude and longitude grid system is likely quite familiar to you, but here is a refresher, pertinent to visualizing the GPS coordinates:

Imaginary lines of latitude—called parallels and approximately 69 miles apart from each other—run horizontally around the globe. The equator is established to be 0°, and each parallel is indicated by degrees from the equator: up to 90°N at the North Pole, and down to 90°S at the South Pole.

Imaginary lines of longitude—called meridians—run perpendicular to latitude lines. Longitude lines are likewise indicated by degrees. Starting from 0° at the Prime Meridian in Greenwich, England, they continue to the east and west until they meet 180° later at the International Date Line in the Pacific Ocean. At the equator, longitude lines also are approximately 69 miles apart, but that distance narrows as the meridians converge toward the North and South Poles.

To convert GPS coordinates given in degrees, minutes, and seconds to the degree–decimal minute format used in this book, the seconds are divided by 60. For more on GPS technology, visit usgs.gov.

Distance and Configuration

Distance notes the length of the hike round-trip, from start to finish. If the hike description includes options to shorten or extend the hike, those round-trip distances will also be factored here. Configuration defines the trail as a loop, an out-and-back (taking you in and out via the same route), a figure eight, or a balloon.

Hiking Time

Distances given are absolute, but hiking times are based on an average hiking speed of 2–3 miles per hour, with time built in for pauses at overlooks and brief rests. Hiking time varies for each hiker, but I like to use the rule of thumb of 3 miles an hour plus an additional hour for every thousand feet of ascent. For trails over 9 miles, I usually add another hour to account for more time to take in the sites and/or a slower pace near the end. Hikers new to the Adirondacks will probably want to pad their time a bit more as they accustom themselves to the more rugged trails.

Highlights

Waterfalls, historic sites, or other features that draw hikers to the trail are emphasized here.

Elevation

In each trail's opener, you will see the elevation at the trailhead and another figure for the peak height on the route. The full hike profile also includes a complete elevation profile (see page 6).

Access

Fees or permits required to hike the trail are detailed here—and noted if there are none. Trail access hours are also shown.

Maps

Resources for maps, in addition to those in this guidebook, are listed here. As previously noted, the publisher and author recommend that you carry more than one map and that you consult those maps before heading out on the trail to resolve any confusion or discrepancy. Common abbreviations listed here include DEC (Department of Environmental Conservation) and USGS (U.S. Geological Survey).

Facilities

This section alerts you to restrooms, phones, water, picnic tables, and other basics at or near the trailhead.

Wheelchair Access

At a glance, you'll see if there are paved sections or other areas for safely using a wheelchair.

Comments

Here you will find assorted nuggets of information, such as whether dogs are allowed on the trails.

Contacts

Listed here are phone numbers and website addresses for checking trail conditions and gleaning other day-to-day information.

Overview, Route Details, and Directions

These three elements provide the main text about the hike. "Overview" gives you a quick summary of what to expect on that trail; the "Route Details" guide you on the hike, start to finish; and "Directions" should get you to the trailhead from a well-known road or highway.

Weather

Weather in the Adirondacks should not be taken lightly. Conditions can change rapidly during all seasons, and the conditions at the base of a tall mountain will certainly not be the same as at the top. When I set out to hike Ampersand Mountain, it was a bright, sunny day in the height of summer. Clouds rolled in, and an unpredicted and severe thunderstorm set in quickly with little warning. Those at the peak sheltered near large boulders at the top, while those at the base turned back. Unfortunately, I was caught in the treeline just below the peak. The situation soon became precarious, as the wind howled and bent trees near the point of snapping. Heavy rains flooded the path, making footing slick. Turning around meant passing through an area where blowdown was likely and unpredictable, and the steep, rocky path became slicker by the minute—hurrying would not be an option. I managed to shelter near the top, where the treeline broke, and descended during a brief break in the weather. When I finally reached my truck, the system had passed, clear skies prevailed, and little evidence of the severe storm remained. Despite raingear, my clothes told a different story than the skies. So as a rule, prepare for the worst case, even if the best is forecasted.

Generally speaking, the Adirondacks are cooler than the rest of New York. This is a welcome respite during summer, but it also means that snow may fall from September into May. Summer temperatures rarely go into the 90s, while winter temperatures often go below zero. Average temperatures are in the mild range, with high 70s typical in summer. Though it varies year to year, the hiking season is generally May–October, though proper attire and preparation is always advised.

Snowshoeing and skiing are also popular in this area, and all but the steepest of the trails described in this book can be done with snowshoes. Indeed, though temperatures often plummet below zero, snowshoeing is often the best way to get some solitude on the more popular trails. Late March and early April, also called the mud season, are likely the least advisable times for hiking in the Adirondacks, and most seasonal roads are closed during this time. Additionally, trail erosion is worst during mud season, and the Department of Environmental Conservation has asked that hikers refrain from hiking in areas above 3,000 feet, as the erosion is particularly damaging to alpine vegetation at this time.

MONTH	HI TEMP	LO TEMP	RAIN OR SNOW
January	27°F	9°F	2.6"
February	31°F	10°F	2.4"
March	41°F	21°F	2.7"
April	55°F	34°F	3.1"
May	68°F	45°F	3.7"
June	76°F	54°F	4.0"
July	81°F	59°F	4.4"
August	78°F	57°F	4.3"
September	71°F	48°F	3.7"
October	58°F	37°F	4.1"
November	45°F	28°F	3.4"
December	33°F	17°F	3.0"

The table on the previous page lists average temperatures and precipitation by month for Adirondack Park. For each month, "Hi Temp" is the average daytime high, "Lo Temp" is the average nighttime low, and "Rain or Snow" is the average precipitation.

Water

With cool temperatures, 3,000 lakes and ponds, and 30,000 miles of streams and rivers, concern for water may seem overly cautious. However *Giardia lamblia,* commonly referred to as giardia, has contaminated many water sources in the Adirondacks. Also known as beaver fever, the intestinal parasite causes—well, put politely—intestinal problems weeks after ingestion, the likes of which most would not wish on their enemies. The words *watery, explosive, foul,* and *rotten* have also been used to describe the aftereffects, so caution is simply necessary. The single-celled organism is transported by all warm-blooded animals, which in turn contaminate water sources. Because beavers are typically in the water and fail to wash their hands, or even leave the water, after using the lavatory, they are often the culprits of the spread and have been rewarded with the disease's moniker. Beavers also abound in the Adirondacks, and many, if not most, streams have beaver activity in or around them. Humans are also culprits in the transporting and contamination of water sources. To prevent contamination, follow the appropriate guidelines for waste disposal as outlined by the Department of Environmental Conservation and as described later in this book (see page 26).

Aside from the inherent risks of drinking untreated water, many of the ponds and lakes are fairly stagnant and taste bad. Effective and proper water treatment is essential for using any source found along the trail. Boiling water for 2–3 minutes is always a safe measure, as are iodine tablets, approved chemical mixes, filtration units rated for giardia, and UV filtration. Some of these methods (such as filtration with an added carbon filter) remove bad tastes, while others add their own taste. My suggestion is to research a filtration method, devise a way to make it palatable, always carry along a means to purify water, and carry enough water for the hike. A cool drink waiting in the car is always a welcome reward, but it's of little use on the trail. Carry a means of purification to help in a pinch or if you underestimate your consumption, but always bring a couple of water bottles for everyone in your group.

How much is enough? Well, one simple physiological fact should convince you to err on the side of excess when deciding how much water to pack: a hiker working hard in 90°F heat needs approximately 10 quarts of fluid per day. That's 2.5 gallons—12 large water bottles or 16 small ones. In other words, pack along one or two bottles even for short hikes. Hydrate prior to your hike, carry (and drink) 6 ounces of water for every mile you plan to hike, and hydrate after the hike.

Clothing

Proper attire will make the difference between enjoying the trail and having a miserable experience. In the worst case it could even save your life. I add these words of caution not to be dramatic but because it is so easy to disregard simple considerations, especially on short trips and especially when it comes to clothing. Weather is unpredictable, trail conditions change or become impassable, we overestimate our abilities and underestimate required hiking times, and wrong turns happen. On a backpacking trip, we are usually prepared for these eventualities because we know that we will be out in the woods for a long time. Don't get me wrong—I'm not advocating hiring a Sherpa or bringing your entire wardrobe, but proper attire at the outset will mitigate most problems.

A few simple guidelines will avert most inconveniences and help you avoid most disasters. When hiking, wear hiking boots and not sandals, flip-flops, or sneakers. Trails in the Adirondacks are hardened, which means they traverse rocky paths to minimize erosion. It protects the forest but is hard on the ankles, so wear

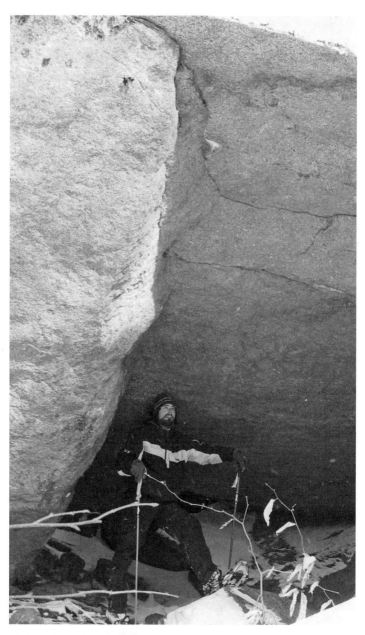

BOULDER CAVE ON THE WAY TO GOOD LUCK CLIFFS *(Trail 2, Good Luck Cliffs, page 35)*

suitable footwear. Proper layering is also essential to comfortable hiking without excessive perspiration, so wear or pack all layers for the season. Dress for the day and prepare for the worst. This means that if it is 75°F and sunny, dress in what is comfortable for you, but bring raingear and do not leave it in the car if the weather looks good. In spring or fall always wear or bring a wool hat and gloves. On the trail I wear pants with zip-off legs and always bring a pack with food and water, as well as a change of socks and shirt, raingear, gaiters, and a warm hat. With these few extra items, you are prepared for any condition or eventuality without adding much weight. In fall, winter, and spring, remember that "cotton kills," so wear silk, wool, or synthetics. In summer cotton may be passable but *only* if you bring a change of clothing that will not get wet. In an emergency you are only prepared with what you have on or with you. Remember, the worst may include spending the night in the woods in spring or fall when daytime and nighttime temperatures vary drastically, so be prepared.

Essential Gear

Along with proper attire, there are several other essential items that every hiker should bring with him or her, even on short day hikes. As I alluded to in the section about clothing, no one plans on a 1-hour hike turning into a night lost in the woods, but it happens all the time to novice and experienced hikers alike. A complete list of items to bring along for day trips and backpacking trips is found in Appendix B (see page 331), but I've listed the essentials here. These items can be carried in your pockets if carefully packed, but carrying a light backpack is often easier. In addition to carrying the items listed below, you need to know how to use them, especially the ones involving navigation.

★   *Water:* Bring a means to carry it and purify it (for example, water bottle and iodine or a filter).

★ *Navigation:* Always carry a map, preferably a topo and a trail map with route description, and a high-quality compass.

★ *Knife or multitool:* A pocketknife and/or multitool with pliers

★ *Light:* A flashlight or headlamp with extra bulb and batteries

★ *Fire:* Windproof matches and/or a lighter, as well as a fire starter

★ *First aid kit:* See below for a list of basic items to be kept in your kit.

★ *Extra food:* Trail mix, granola bars, or other high-energy foods

★ *Extra clothes:* Raingear, warm hat, gloves, and a change of socks and shirt

★ *Sun protection:* Sunglasses, lip balm, sunblock, and a sun hat

First Aid Kit

A typical first aid kit may contain more items than you might think necessary. These are just the basics. Prepackaged kits in waterproof bags are available. Even though quite a few items are listed here, they pack down into a small space.

★ Adhesive bandages

★ Antibiotic ointment (Neosporin or the generic equivalent)

★ Athletic tape

★ Benadryl or the generic equivalent, diphenhydramine (in case of allergic reactions)

★ Blister kit (such as moleskin or Spenco 2nd Skin)

★ Butterfly-closure bandages

★ Elastic bandages or joint wraps

★ Epinephrine in a prefilled syringe (for people known to have severe allergic reactions to such things as bee stings, usually by prescription only)

★ Gauze and compress pads (one roll and a half dozen 4-by-4-inch pads)

★ Hydrogen peroxide or iodine

★ Ibuprofen or acetaminophen

★ Insect repellent

★ Matches or a pocket lighter

★ Sunscreen

★ Tweezers

★ Whistle (more effective at signaling rescuers than your voice)

General Safety

To some potential mountain enthusiasts, the deep woods seem inordinately dark and perilous. It is the fear of the unknown that causes this anxiety. No doubt, potentially dangerous situations can occur outdoors, but as long as you use sound judgment and prepare yourself before hitting the trail, you'll be much safer in the woods than in most urban areas of the country. It is better to look at a backcountry hike as a fascinating chance to discover the unknown rather than a chance for potential disaster. If you're new to the game, I suggest starting out easy and finding a person who knows more to help you out. In addition, here are a few tips to make your trip safer and easier.

★ *Always let someone know your plans in advance.* Tell your safety person which trails you will be on, when and where you expect to depart from, and when and where you expect to return. Though you are primarily responsible for your safety, your safety person is your backup plan and will alert rescuers where to look for you. Remember to tell your safety person all changes in your plans and check in to let him or her know your trip went well.

★ *Always sign in and out of the trail registers provided.* If you are hiking several trails, it will alert rescuers where you are and, sometimes more important, where you are not.

While getting lost is unlikely on shorter trails, injury is a distinct possibility, as indicated by numerous warning signs of precipitous cliffs. While bravado may foolishly deter people from using the registers for the first reason, the following reason may appeal more to their self-interest. The Department of Environmental Conservation and the state base many of their trail-maintenance and funding decisions on trail registers. So if you want to see your favorite trails maintained or want more like them, then let the registers act as your democratic voice in the wilderness.

★ *Never rely on a cell phone, but bring one just in case.* Reception is spotty at best and virtually nonexistent in most areas—and your phone won't work as kindling.

★ *Always carry food and water,* whether you are planning to go overnight or not. Food will give you energy, help keep you warm, and sustain you in an emergency until help arrives. You never know if a stream will be nearby when you become thirsty. Bring potable water or treat water before drinking it from a stream. Boil or filter all found water before drinking it.

★ *Stay on designated trails.* Most hikers get lost when they leave the path. Even on the most clearly marked trails, there is usually a point where you have to stop and consider what direction to head. If you become disoriented, don't panic. As soon as you think that you may be off track, stop, assess your current direction, and then retrace your steps to the point where you went astray. Using a map, a compass, and this book, and keeping in mind what you have passed thus far, reorient yourself and trust your judgment on which way to continue. If you become absolutely unsure of how to continue, return to your vehicle the way you came in. Should you become completely lost and have no idea how to return to the trailhead, remaining in place along the trail and waiting for help is most often the best option for adults and always the best option for children.

★ *Be especially careful when crossing streams.* Whether you are fording the stream or crossing on a log, make every step count. If you have any doubt about maintaining your balance on a log, ford the stream instead. When crossing, use a trekking pole or stout stick for balance and face upstream as you cross. If a stream seems too deep to ford, turn back. Whatever is on the other side is not worth risking your life.

★ *Be careful at overlooks.* While these areas may provide spectacular views, they are potentially hazardous. Stay back from the edge of outcrops and be absolutely sure of your footing; a misstep can mean a nasty and possibly fatal fall.

★ *Standing dead trees and storm-damaged living trees* pose a real hazard to hikers and tent campers. These trees may have loose or broken limbs that could fall at any time. When choosing a spot to rest or a backcountry campsite, look up.

★ *Know the symptoms of hypothermia.* Shivering and forgetfulness are the two most common indicators of this stealthy killer. Hypothermia can occur at any elevation, even in the summer, especially when the hiker is wearing lightweight cotton clothing. If symptoms arise, get the victim shelter, hot liquids, and dry clothes or a dry sleeping bag.

★ *Take along your brain.* A cool, calculating mind is the single most important asset on the trail. Think before you act. Watch your step. Plan ahead. Avoiding accidents is the best way to ensure a rewarding and relaxing hike.

★ *Ask questions.* State forest and park employees are there to help. It's a lot easier to ask advice beforehand, and it will help you avoid a mishap away from civilization when it's too late to amend an error.

Animal, Insect, and Plant Hazards

BLACK BEARS Black bears are found throughout New York state but are most frequently encountered in the Adirondacks and occasionally in the Catskills. Though attacks by black bears are virtually unheard of, a bear tearing up your gear or rummaging about outside your tent will give anyone a start. If you encounter a bear at your campsite or while hiking, remain calm and never run away. Make loud noises to scare off the bear and back away slowly.

Black bears normally avoid humans, but you should always leave them an escape route if you encounter them. They can sprint up to 35 miles per hour and are strong swimmers and great tree climbers.

In primitive and remote areas, assume that bears are present; in more developed sites, ask the park staff about the current bear situation. Most encounters are food related, as bears have an exceptional sense of smell and will eat anything. A clean site, combined with care and caution, will keep these foragers away from your campsite. Store all food, cooking equipment, and garbage in tightly sealed containers and place well away from your tent. In remote areas or those with recent bear activity, store all items in storage lockers or bear canisters, or suspend them in a sack 12 feet above the ground, 6 feet below branches, and 12 feet from neighboring trees. Make sure that your site is clean, and never leave food unattended. Wash utensils and cooking equipment at least 100 feet from your site, and never dump uneaten food on the ground. Do not bring food into your tent, and do not sleep in clothes worn while preparing food. Never leave scented products of any kind—food, beverages, or personal-care products, such as lotion or sunscreen—in your vehicle or unattended in the park area. Generally, proper food preparation and garbage disposal will help maintain a pristine wilderness, the safety of bears and other wildlife, and an enjoyable camping experience for everyone. For updated information and rules regarding acceptable bear canisters (required for overnight trips in the Eastern High Peaks Wilderness area), see the Department of Environmental Conservation website: www.dec.ny.gov/animals/7225.html.

RATTLESNAKES New York has a variety of snakes—including garter, milk, and water snakes—most of which are benign. Timber rattlesnakes, northern copperheads, and eastern massasauga rattlesnakes are the exceptions, though they primarily dwell in very isolated areas.

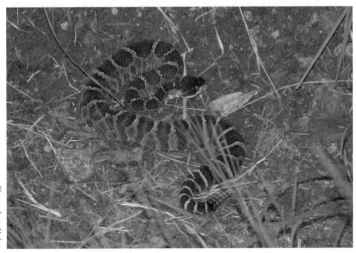

Photo: Jane Huber

According to the Department of Environmental Conservation, the massasauga is found in two isolated marshy areas: one near Syracuse and the other near Rochester. The copperhead is found mostly along the Hudson Valley but is largely absent from the Catskills. Timber rattlesnakes are the most widely dispersed of the three and are found in rugged deciduous forests along the southern edge of the state and up into the eastern Adirondacks. Encounters with any of these species are very rare.

When hiking, stick to well-used trails and wear over-the-ankle boots and loose-fitting, long pants. Rattlesnakes like to bask in the sun and won't bite unless threatened. Do not step or put your hands where you cannot see, and avoid wandering around in the dark. Step *on* logs and rocks, never over them, and be especially careful when climbing rocks or gathering firewood. Always avoid walking through dense brush or willow thickets. Keep in mind that rattlers want to avoid confrontation and generally will alert you if you wander too close for their comfort. Hibernation season is October–April.

The only known treatment for a snakebite is intravenous antivenom, only available at a hospital. If you are hiking alone and get bitten, calmly walk to where you can get help. If someone in your group has been bitten, send another person to get help quickly while the victim rests.

MOSQUITOES You will encounter mosquitoes on most of the hikes described in this book. Insect repellent and/or repellent-impregnated clothing are the only simple methods to ward off these pests. Mosquitoes in New York are known to carry the West Nile virus, so all due caution should be taken to avoid mosquito bites.

BLACK FLIES Though certainly a pest and maddening annoyance, the worst a black fly will cause is an itchy welt. They are most active mid-May–June, during the day, and especially before thunderstorms, as well as during the morning and evening hours. Insect repellent has some effect, though the only way to keep them from swarming is to keep moving.

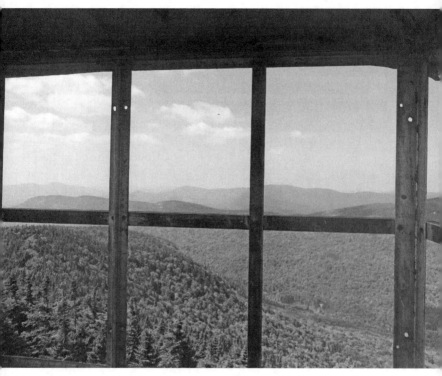

INSIDE THE FIRE TOWER ON TOP OF SNOWY MOUNTAIN *(Trail 18, Snowy Mountain, page 129)*

TICKS Ticks are often found on brush and tall grass, waiting to hitch a ride on a warm-blooded passerby. Adult ticks are most active in New York between April and May and again between October and November. Among the local varieties of ticks, the black-legged tick, commonly called the deer tick, is the primary carrier of Lyme disease. Several strategies reduce the chances of ticks getting under your skin. Some people choose to wear light-colored clothing, so ticks can be spotted before they make it to the skin. Most important, be sure to visually check your hair, back of neck, armpits, and socks at the end of the hike. During your posthike shower, take a moment to do a more complete body check. For ticks that are already embedded, grasp the tick as close to the skin's surface as possible with tweezers, and pull upward with steady, even pressure. Do not puncture a tick, as this might release harmful bacteria. Use disinfectant solution on the wound.

POISON IVY, OAK, AND SUMAC Recognizing and avoiding poison ivy, oak, and sumac are the most effective ways to prevent the painful, itchy rashes associated with these plants. Poison ivy occurs as a vine or ground cover, 3 leaflets to a leaf; poison oak occurs as either a vine or shrub, also with 3 leaflets; and poison sumac flourishes in swampland, each leaf having 7–13 leaflets. Urushiol, the oil in the sap of these plants, is responsible for the rash. Within 14 hours of exposure, raised lines and/or blisters will appear on the affected area, accompanied by a terrible itch. Refrain from scratching because bacteria under your fingernails can cause an infection. Wash and dry the rash thoroughly, applying a calamine lotion to help dry out the rash. If itching or blistering is severe, seek medical attention. If you do come into contact with one of these plants, remember that oil-contaminated clothes, pets, or gear can easily cause an irritating rash on you or someone else, so wash not only any exposed parts of your body but also clothes, gear, and pets, if applicable.

Hunting

Unlike many national and state parks, hunting is allowed in Adirondack Park. Separate rules, regulations, and licenses govern the various hunting types and related seasons. Though there are generally no problems, hikers may wish to forgo their trips during the big-game seasons, when the woods suddenly seem filled with orange and camouflage. The following is a list of big-game seasons.

★ *Early bear season:* The first Saturday after the second Monday in September; lasts four weeks

★ *Archery season (deer and bear):* September 27 to opening of regular season

★ *Muzzle-loading season:* Seven days prior to regular season

★ *Regular season:* Next-to-last Saturday in October through the first Sunday in December

Tips for Enjoying Adirondack Park

One of the best features of Adirondack Park is its democratic nature. It is meant for the public to enjoy its wild character and is open to all. There are few if any fees, permits, or licenses required for this enjoyment—and none for those who simply wish to hike the trails. Simply drive to your trailhead, get out of your car, and hit the trail. It is a luxury and a responsibility. Without park staff cleaning, maintaining, and policing the way they typically do in other parks, the burden for cleanliness, maintenance, and your own safety lies on your own shoulders. Practicing the ethos of carry-in and carry-out will ensure that other hikers enjoy the wilderness as much as, and in the same way, you have. By maintaining campsites, lean-tos, and fire rings, you will ensure others get to enjoy them and find them useful too. Avoiding destructive behavior, such as chopping down trees for firewood or causing unnecessary erosion by taking shortcuts, means the forever-wild character of the Adirondacks will remain.

Backcountry Advice and DEC Regulations

The entire park lies under the jurisdiction of the Department of Environmental Conservation (DEC), and its rules and regulations regarding hiking and backcountry camping apply for all state lands within the park. Camping is permitted within the forest preserve without a permit as long as you follow the regulations below. The DEC's rules and regulations are essentially the same sound, safe, and practical advice I would offer, so I recap them below.

★ *Camping is prohibited within 150 feet of any road,* trail, spring, stream, pond, or other body of water, except at areas designated by a CAMP HERE disk.

★ *Groups of 10 or more persons* or stays of more than three days in one place require a permit from the New York state forest ranger responsible for the area.

★ *Lean-tos are available in many areas* on a first-come, first-serve basis. Lean-tos cannot be used exclusively and must be shared with other campers.

★ *Use pit privies provided near popular camping areas* and trailheads. If none are available, dispose of human waste by digging a hole 6–8 inches deep at least 150 feet from water or campsites. Cover with leaves and soil.

★ *Do not use soap to wash yourself,* clothing, or dishes within 150 feet of water.

★ *Drinking and cooking water should be boiled* for 5 minutes, treated with purifying tablets, or filtered through a filtration device to prevent instances of giardia infection.

★ *Fires should be built in existing fire pits or fireplaces* if provided. Use only dead and down wood for fires. Cutting standing trees is prohibited. Extinguish all fires with water, and stir ashes until they are cold to the touch. Do not build fires in areas marked by a NO FIRES disk. Camp stoves are safer, more efficient, and cleaner.

★ *Carry out what you carry in.* Practice Leave No Trace camping and hiking guidelines.

★ *Keep your pet under control.* Restrain it on a leash when others approach. Collect and bury droppings away from water, trails, and campsites. Keep your pet away from drinking-water sources.

★ *Observe and enjoy wildlife and plants,* but leave them undisturbed.

★ *Removing plants, rocks, fossils, or artifacts* from state land without a permit is illegal.

★ *Except in an emergency,* or between December 15 and April 30, camping is prohibited above an elevation of 4,000 feet in the Adirondacks.

★ *At all times, only emergency fires are permitted* above 4,000 feet in the Adirondacks.

Trail Etiquette

Whether you're on a city, county, state, or national park trail, always remember that great care and resources (from nature as well as from your tax dollars) have gone into creating these trails. Treat the trail, wildlife, and fellow hikers with respect.

★ *Hike on open trails only.* Respect trail and road closures (ask if not sure), avoid possible trespassing on private land, and obtain all permits and authorization as required. Also, leave gates as you found them or as marked.

★ *Leave only footprints.* Be sensitive to the ground beneath you. Stay on existing trails rather than blazing new ones. Pack out what you pack in. No one likes to see the trash someone else has left behind.

★ *Never spook animals.* An unannounced approach, a sudden movement, or a loud noise startles most animals. Surprised animals can be dangerous to you, to others, and to themselves. Give them extra room and time to adjust to your presence.

★ *Observe the yield signs* that are displayed around the region's trailheads and backcountry. They advise that hikers yield to horses, and bikers yield to both horses and hikers. A common courtesy on hills is that hikers and bikers yield to any uphill traffic.

★ *When encountering mounted riders or horse packers,* hikers can courteously step off the trail, on the downhill side, if possible. Speak to the riders before they reach you and do not hide behind trees. You are less spooky if the horse can see and hear you. Resist the urge to pet or touch the horses unless you are invited to do so.

★ *Plan ahead.* Know your equipment, your ability, and the area in which you are hiking—and prepare accordingly. Be self-sufficient at all times; carry necessary supplies for changes in weather or other conditions. A well-executed trip is satisfying.

★ *Be courteous to other hikers, bikers, equestrians,* and others you encounter on the trails.

Southern (Hikes 1–7)

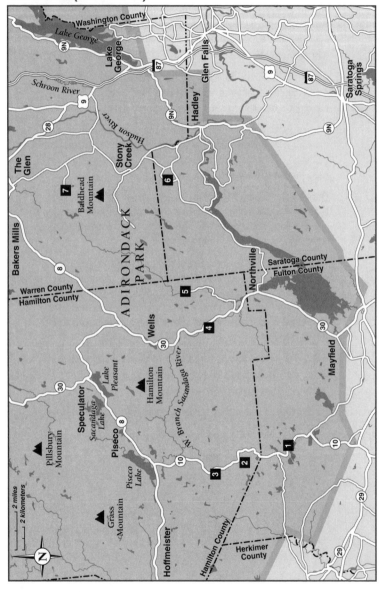

Southern

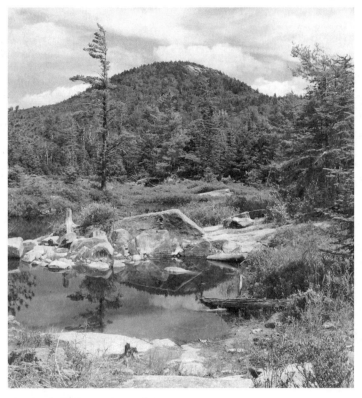

CRANE MOUNTAIN *(Trail 7, page 61)*

Stewart and Indian Lakes

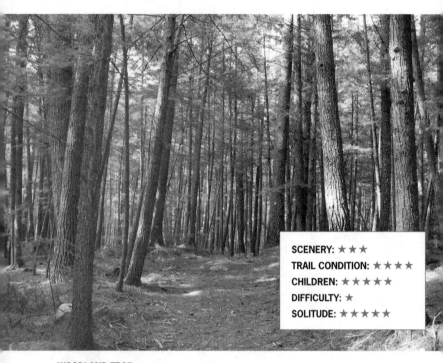

SCENERY: ★ ★ ★
TRAIL CONDITION: ★ ★ ★ ★
CHILDREN: ★ ★ ★ ★ ★
DIFFICULTY: ★
SOLITUDE: ★ ★ ★ ★ ★

WOODLAND TRAIL

GPS COORDINATES: N43° 10.790'   W74° 30.295'

DISTANCE & CONFIGURATION: 4.6-mile out-and-back

HIKING TIME: 2–3 hours

HIGHLIGHTS: Two secluded lakes

ELEVATION: 1,603' at trailhead, 2,044' at highest point

ACCESS: Open 24/7; no fees or permits required

MAPS: National Geographic *Adirondack Park, Northville/Raquette Lake* (#744)

FACILITIES: None

WHEELCHAIR ACCESS: No

CONTACTS: Central and Southern Adirondack trail information: www.dec.ny.gov/outdoor /9200.html; emergency contact: 518-891-0235

Overview

This easy hike is a great destination for people who wish to explore two remote, picturesque lakes for fishing or a picnic. With a few moderate climbs, it is a good trail for children, and wildlife viewing at both lakes provides additional interest.

Route Details

Located in the Shaker Mountain Wild Forest, the trail uses old logging roads, so the grades are mostly gentle and easily accessible to hikers of all experience levels. The area had been heavily logged before state acquisitions, and much of the forest is still in a phase of regeneration. However, the acquisitions occurred decades ago, and traces of past logging have disappeared. Wild forest areas—in contrast to wilderness, primitive, or canoe areas—are considered less ecologically fragile, allowing for a greater variety of uses and more intensive activities. Don't let the distinction fool you, though, as they are definitely wild places and provide excellent wilderness experiences. Access to the parking area is at the left fork along Green Lake Road, which appears to be little more than a driveway. The well-maintained and spacious lot provides parking for the Kane Mountain Trail as well, but it can easily accommodate a dozen cars, so space should not be a concern.

The trail begins to the right of the trail register on the north end of the parking lot. Shrouded in tall pines, it follows an access road to a small fish hatchery created by the damming of Otter Lake's outlet, and you can hear water spilling over the concrete dam in most seasons. The trail diverges from the road shortly before the pond on your right. The exact path may be a little hard to discern, but a wooden bridge and a sign prohibiting the use of baitfish will steer you.

A note to anglers: The Department of Environmental Conservation has gone to great lengths to reestablish native brook trout and the endangered round whitefish in some of the isolated waters of the Adirondacks. Reestablishment methods vary but include treating entire lakes with rotenone to remove competing, nonnative species

Stewart and Indian Lakes

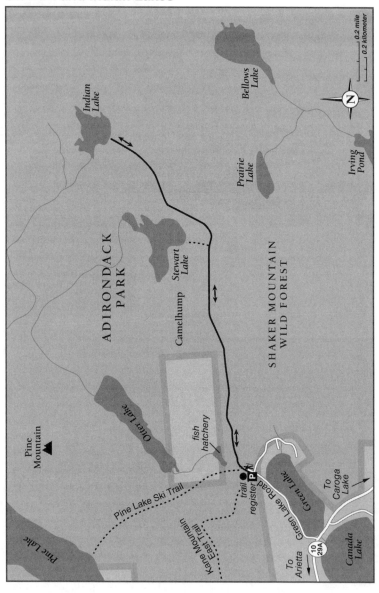

and then restocking the waters with native fish. Due to the physical characteristics of the various Adirondack waterways, the success of this technique is limited and expensive. When the technique is successful, those same physical characteristics mean there will be lasting success and that native fish populations can thrive. Unfortunately, the reintroduction of nonnative species is almost exclusively a consequence of the unintentional release of baitfish by anglers into the reestablished ecosystems. So leave the bait bucket at home when visiting the prized fishing waters of the Adirondacks.

Once on the trail, you will notice that it is emblazoned by yellow trail markers and very easy to follow the rest of the way. A quick climb takes you along a low ridge overlooking the pond to your left. The trail climbs through a mixed hardwood forest dominated by birch and beech trees. The grade is very moderate for the first 0.7 mile, at which point you encounter a muddy area. The trail climbs more steeply after this muddy area, but at approximately 1.2 miles it levels off to a more gently rolling terrain. Farther along the trail, the forest canopy gets higher and the understory thins, allowing deeper views into the surrounding forest. You catch glimpses of Stewart Lake as you approach 1.3 miles, where there is a fork in the trail. The main

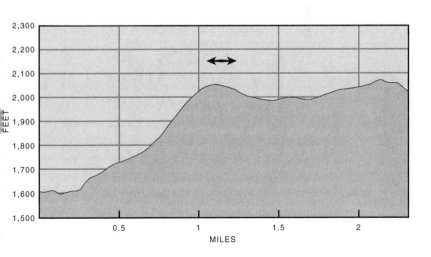

trail continues on the right toward Indian Lake, while the left fork takes you through a stand of pine and hemlock to a boggy area that surrounds Stewart Lake. The marshland prevents you from gaining direct access to the lake but makes for good wildlife viewing.

Back along the trail, you encounter some mucky areas that you will have to negotiate on your own, as no good way bypasses the muck. At 2 miles, you pass a thick carpet of club moss, which at first glance looks like tree saplings but is actually more closely related to ferns. At this point, you begin the descent to Indian Lake, where the trail ends at the shore. A path to the left follows the shoreline toward a rock that juts out into the lake and provides additional vantage points. The remote setting promises a wonderful opportunity to view a variety of wildlife, including a beaver lodge.

Directions

From the southern intersection of NY 10 and NY 29A in downtown Caroga Lake, head north on NY 10/NY 29A. At 3.4 miles past the intersection, turn right onto Green Lake Road.

From the intersection of NY 8 and NY 10 in Piseco, head 19.6 miles south on NY 10, and turn left (1.9 miles past the northern intersection of NY 10 and NY 29A near Pine Lake Park) onto Green Lake Road. Follow Green Lake Road north along the west edge of the shore. At 0.5 mile, bear left onto the parking area drive.

Good Luck Cliffs

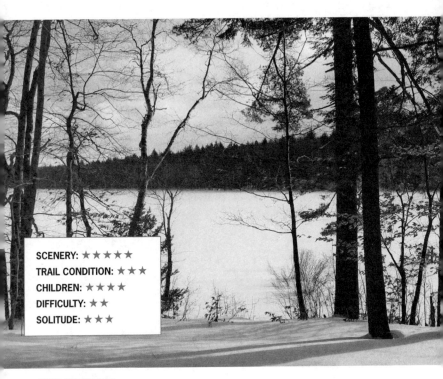

SCENERY: ★ ★ ★ ★ ★
TRAIL CONDITION: ★ ★ ★
CHILDREN: ★ ★ ★ ★
DIFFICULTY: ★ ★
SOLITUDE: ★ ★ ★

GOOD LUCK LAKE

GPS COORDINATES: N43° 15.352'   W74° 32.292'

DISTANCE & CONFIGURATION: 3.4-mile out-and-back

HIKING TIME: 2–3 hours

HIGHLIGHTS: Dramatic cliffs, panoramic views

ELEVATION: 1,693' at trailhead, 2,284' at highest point

ACCESS: Open 24/7; no fees or permits required

MAPS: National Geographic *Adirondack Park, Northville/Raquette Lake* (#744)

FACILITIES: None

WHEELCHAIR ACCESS: No

CONTACTS: Central and Southern Adirondack trail information: www.dec.ny.gov/outdoor
/9200.html; emergency contact: 518-891-0235

Good Luck Cliffs

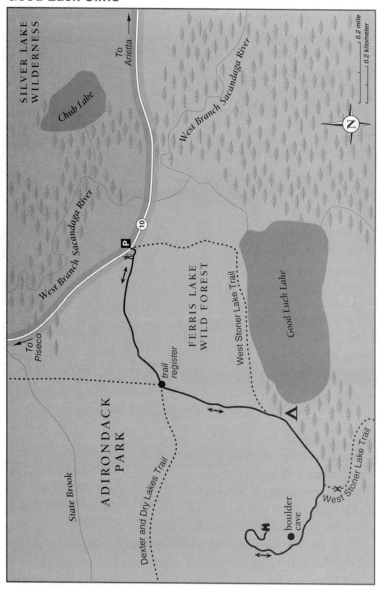

Overview

Sheer cliffs are almost standard in the High Peaks region, but in the southern foothills, these dramatic cliffs are unique and rival those anywhere in the Adirondacks. Though the path to Good Luck Cliffs is technically a bushwhack, the cliffs are frequented enough that even in the height of winter, you can find your way to the mountaintop.

Route Details

The parking area is a few hundred yards north of the second bridge that crosses the West Branch of the Sacandaga River along NY 10 in the town of Arietta. Coming from the south, the parking area is a large pulloff on the right-hand side of the road.

The trailhead is across the street and has signs indicating that Dexter Lake is 4.1 miles, Potter Homestead is 7.1 miles, and Good Luck Lake is 0.4 mile, though the latter is along a separate trail. The trail register is approximately 0.5 mile ahead at a trail junction. Follow the snowmobile and red trail disks west along mostly level terrain. Shortly after passing through a wet section, you reach the trail register and junction with other trails. To the right is a snowmobile trail that

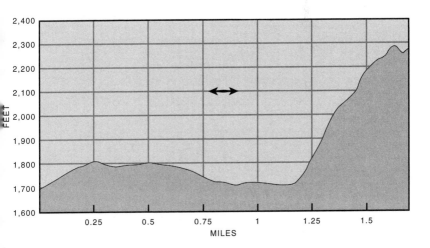

parallels NY 10. Straight ahead is the trail to Dry and Dexter Lakes, 1.6 and 2.4 miles respectively. The left trail takes you to the west shore of Good Luck Lake (including some tent sites), Spectacle Lake, and the unmarked path to the cliffs and Good Luck Mountain summit.

The trail has several muddy and wet sections as you make your way south toward the lake, and it even shares space with a stream for a while. The trail begins to descend from this junction, and at approximately 1 mile in, the lake comes into view. A designated campsite to the left of the trail offers a great view of the lake. The cliffs soon become visible, looming off to your right, and you continue past the western tip of the lake through a marshy area, where the evergreens become denser. After crossing a short bridge, you reach the crest of a tiny hill, at 1.3 miles, below which is another bridge that crosses a stream that feeds Good Luck Lake. To your right is the unmarked path that leads to the cliffs.

The path parallels the feeder stream briefly on your left, along an elevated knoll, before swinging northwest toward the cliffs. Shortly after, the trail climbs and you rock-hop across a stream that cuts the gorge along the cliff's southwest face. The path follows within a few hundred feet of this stream all the way to a notch that lies just below the cliffs. In winter, icicles form sheets of ice along the southern tumble of boulders, creating an amazing winter wonderland setting.

Though the cliffs have been visible through most of the climb, their full grandeur is not fully expressed until you reach the small saddle beneath the west face of the cliff. The trail swings north here, and you will navigate your way around a jumble of boulders that covers the valley floor. The huge boulders provide an opportunity for exploration, including many small caves that are formed in the mass of rock. You pass a noteworthy cave on the right at 1.4 miles.

You probably have heard the stream flowing on your right, and at 1.5 miles, you recross it before the final ascent to the clifftop. The trail is much steeper and the path less distinct, but as long as you keep the cliffs to your right, you will eventually make your way to the north, or back, side of the cliffs. About 0.1 mile from the

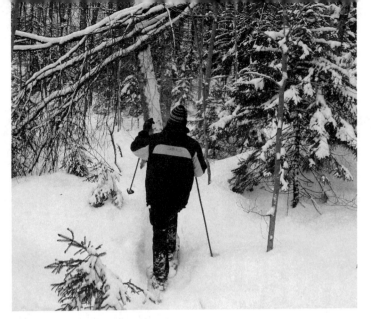

SNOWSHOEING ALONG THE UNMARKED PART OF THE TRAIL

stream crossing, you reach a fork in the trail in a stand of spruce trees. To the left is a slight northward jog in the trail that leads to the clifftop, while the right trail leads to the clifftop a little more steeply but more directly. Either way, you reach the top shortly; from there, take any of the numerous paths that weave their way from outlook to outlook. Along the southwest edge is a particularly amazing vista that shows expansive views down to the valley, with Spectacle Lake in the foreground.

Directions

FROM THE SOUTH   From the intersection of NY 29A and NY 10, north of Caroga Lake near Pine Lake Park, head 6 miles north on NY 10. The large parking area is on the right just past the second bridge crossing the Sacandaga River in the town of Arietta.

FROM THE NORTH   From the intersection of NY 8 and NY 10 in Piseco, head 11.6 miles south on NY 10. The large parking area is on your left.

Jockeybush Lake

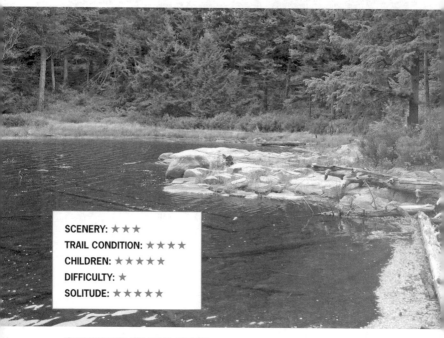

SCENERY: ★ ★ ★
TRAIL CONDITION: ★ ★ ★ ★
CHILDREN: ★ ★ ★ ★ ★
DIFFICULTY: ★
SOLITUDE: ★ ★ ★ ★ ★

JOCKEYBUSH LAKE NEAR OUTLET

GPS COORDINATES: N43° 18.057'   W74° 33.905'

DISTANCE & CONFIGURATION: 2.3-mile out-and-back

HIKING TIME: 2 hours

HIGHLIGHTS: Pristine lake, waterfall

ELEVATION: 1,755' at trailhead, 1,964' at highest point

ACCESS: Open 24/7; no fees or permits required

MAPS: National Geographic *Adirondack Park, Northville/Raquette Lake* (#744)

FACILITIES: None

WHEELCHAIR ACCESS: No

COMMENTS: During the spring thaw, Jockeybush Outlet may require wading, so plan accordingly.

CONTACTS: Central and Southern Adirondack trail information: www.dec.ny.gov/outdoor /9200.html; emergency contact: 518-891-0235

Overview

Another one of the short hikes featured in the book, Jockeybush Lake promises a varied experience, from streamside hiking and stream crossings to lakeside camping and even a small waterfall. As with other short hikes, this one promises a great experience for beginning hikers and a pleasant trip for the whole family.

Route Details

Parking for Jockeybush Lake is a pulloff on the west side of NY 10, just across from Lake Alma. Essentially a pond, Lake Alma has a large painted sign with a green pine tree that is clearly visible when approaching from the south. Coming from the north, keep an eye out for the Department of Environmental Conservation trail signs.

The trail begins in the northwest corner of the pulloff, and the trail register is a few yards along the path. The trail is well marked with blue trail disks and has no intersections, so finding your way is straightforward. Roughly 0.3 mile in, you cross a seasonal stream that has a few mucky spots, and you will likely have to find a crossing off the trail. You will soon see Jockeybush Outlet flowing on your left and will cross to its southern bank across a rocky wash. During summer this crossing will barely break your stride, but during times of high water, you may have to wade. Shortly after crossing the outlet, you pass a small waterfall on your right that feeds into the outlet. The cascade weaves its way down moss-covered ledges into a verdant jumble of rocks. You can rock-hop around and eventually scramble to the top of the cascade some dozen feet above the outlet to see another tiny cascade.

After the short diversion at the falls, the trail weaves its way along the southern banks of the outlet for the rest of the way to Jockeybush Lake, almost without incident. The one exception is a long muddy section, about a mile in, that fills the entire trail. You'll have to either traverse the muck or bypass along one of the newer footpaths that hikers have made. As is the case with most trails, it is

Jockeybush Lake

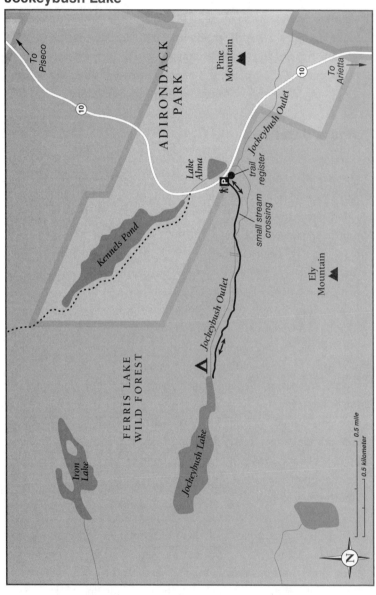

Pine Mountain

To Piseco

To Arietta

ADIRONDACK PARK

Jockeybush Outlet

10

10

Lake Alma

trail register

small stream crossing

Kennels Pond

Ely Mountain

Jockeybush Outlet

FERRIS LAKE WILD FOREST

Jockeybush Lake

Iron Lake

0.5 mile

0.5 kilometer

N

best to minimize your impact on the surrounding forest by following a path already worn by previous hikers than tramping on undisturbed areas. Soon after the mire, you will find yourself on the eastern end of Jockeybush Lake. The lake is deep, as far as Adirondack lakes are concerned, but it's not readily apparent at this end as it is shallow here. Bushwhacks along either shore reveal that the lake is deeper than it first appears. At this end of the lake, a logjam forms a dam, as well as a means to the opposite bank of the outlet, where a designated campsite is situated in a small stand of hemlocks. The campsite has admirable views west along the fingerlike lake and is an ideal spot to picnic during a day trip. Numerous footpaths diverge from the end of the trailhead and campsite, promising other vantage points and even a prime swimming spot, but the trail described ends here. Return the way you came for a round-trip of 2.3 miles.

Directions

FROM THE SOUTH   From the intersection of NY 29A and NY 10, north of Caroga Lake near Pine Lake Park, head 9.6 miles north on NY 10. The parking area is on the left, opposite Lake Alma, and has a large brown-and-white sign.

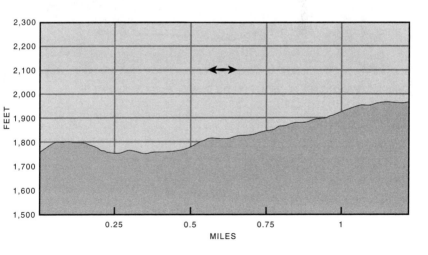

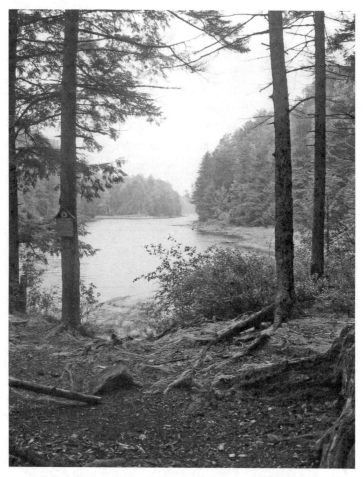

JOCKEYBUSH LAKE AS SEEN FROM THE CAMPSITE ON ITS EASTERN TIP

FROM THE NORTH   From the intersection of NY 8 and NY 10 in Piseco, head 7.9 miles south on NY 10. The parking area is on your right, opposite Lake Alma.

Groff Creek

SCENERY: ★ ★ ★	
TRAIL CONDITION: ★ ★ ★	
CHILDREN: ★ ★ ★	
DIFFICULTY: ★	
SOLITUDE: ★ ★ ★ ★ ★	

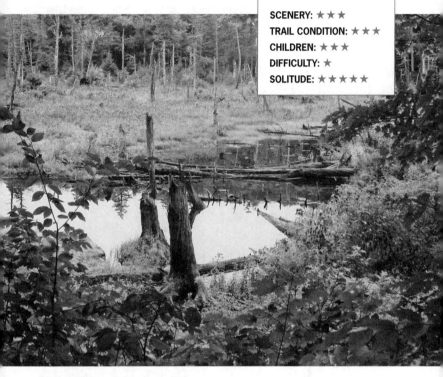

UPPER PORTION OF GROFF CREEK

GPS COORDINATES: N43° 18.823'   W74° 15.402'

DISTANCE & CONFIGURATION: 5.0-mile out-and-back

HIKING TIME: 3–4 hours

HIGHLIGHTS: Two unique waterfalls

ELEVATION: 918' at trailhead, 1,322' at highest point

ACCESS: Open 24/7; no fees or permits required

MAPS: National Geographic *Adirondack Park, Northville/Raquette Lake* (#744)

FACILITIES: None

WHEELCHAIR ACCESS: No

CONTACTS: Silver Lake Wilderness: www.dec.ny.gov/lands/100874.html; Central and Southern Adirondack trail information: www.dec.ny.gov/outdoor/9200.html; emergency contact: 518-891-0235

Groff Creek

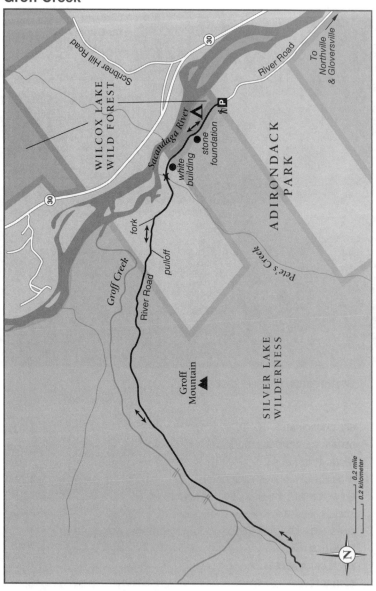

Overview

The two unique waterfalls along Groff Creek make this a must-experience trip for waterfall lovers. Though technically a bushwhack (the trail is unmarked), it is very easy to follow all the way to the marsh at the end.

Route Details

The trail is at the end of the maintained section of River Road. The trail continues along this road briefly, but a sign warns that the road farther on is abandoned and you are proceeding at your own risk. Park along the pullout to the west of this sign, and make your way north along the broad, flat road. The road parallels and provides pleasant views of the Sacandaga River. At 0.2 mile, you will pass a designated camping area on your right that is encircled by tall pines and provides ample room to set up. Views of the river are limited from this site. Shortly past the designated campsite, you will see the remains of an old stone foundation on your left. A little more than 0.3 mile along the road, pass the posts for an old vehicle barrier and then a small white building on your left. A wooden bridge crosses

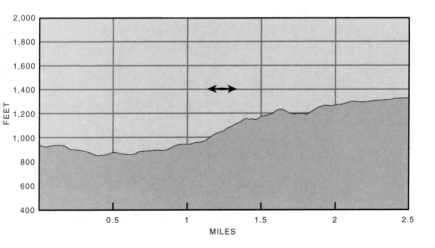

Pete's Creek just past this building. Approximately 0.3 mile after the bridge, you reach an intersection in the road. Continue straight on the right-hand side of the fork another 0.1 mile, where you reach Forest Preserve lands.

You will pass a pulloff along the road on your left and then a small parking area at 0.8 mile. This marks the end of the road and the farthest point reached by vehicle if you should chance the abandoned road. The trail to your left still follows an old logging road, but nature has reclaimed much of it, and only a narrow footpath remains. The trail begins to climb for the next 0.5 mile as you work your way to the north side of Groff Mountain. The terrain falls off steeply on your right down to Groff Creek, and about 1.8 miles from the start, you will glimpse the first waterfall along the creek. There is no clear path down to view the waterfall, so pick your way carefully down the hillside and through the tall hemlocks to the top of the falls. The banks of the creek surrounding the waterfall are extremely steep on this side, but if you make your way to the top of the falls, you can cross to the other side and then zigzag your way down to the base. The nearly 30-foot vertical drop ends in a shallow pool, which is surrounded on three sides with vertical walls. Inside this natural amphitheater, the tumble of the falls drowns out all other sounds.

The second waterfall along this section of the creek is 0.1 mile farther west along the trail. Unlike the previous waterfall, this one is visible from the trail. Similar to the first one, no distinguishable path leads to it, though the route down is less steep. A frothy cascade, this waterfall steps its way down a series of ledges to a shallow pool as well. Downstream are a series of flumes and cascades that add waterscapes of their own.

While exploring these falls, you are in prime habitat of the red-spotted newt. The adult newt is olive green with red spots along its back, but you are far more likely to encounter and recognize it in its terrestrial juvenile stage. The juvenile, known as a red eft, is brilliant orange with red dots and is common in woodlands near creeks and streams.

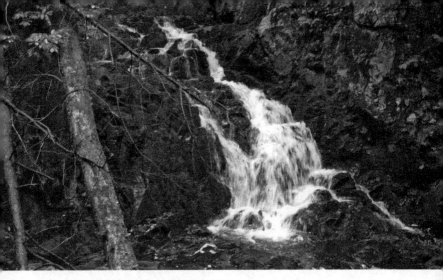

SECOND WATERFALL ALONG GROFF CREEK

The trail continues another 0.5 mile west to where the creek levels off and a marsh forms. It continues along the south side of the marsh, though where it truly ends is hard to discern. Another set of waterfalls is said to be found on the opposite shore if you follow a tributary stream around a major bend. This would require serious bushwhacking, as there is no clear path. I attempted to find them during a heavy rain but soon decided to leave their discovery for another expedition. Return back along the path for a total trip length of 5 miles.

Directions

FROM THE SOUTH   From the intersection of NY 30 and NY 30A in Gloversville, head 13.6 miles north on NY 30, and turn left onto County Road 6/Benson Road. Within a couple hundred feet, turn right onto River Road. Follow River Road north 4.6 miles to where the signs warn that the road is abandoned. Park to the left of the road.

FROM THE NORTH   From the intersection of NY 30 and NY 8 in Wells, head 15.8 miles south on NY 30, and turn right onto CR 6/Benson Road. Within a couple hundred feet, turn right onto River Road. Follow River Road north 4.6 miles to where the signs warn that the road is abandoned. Park to the left of the road.

Tenant Creek Falls

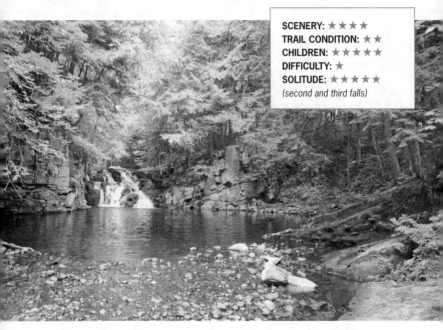

SCENERY: ★ ★ ★ ★
TRAIL CONDITION: ★ ★
CHILDREN: ★ ★ ★ ★ ★
DIFFICULTY: ★
SOLITUDE: ★ ★ ★ ★ ★
(second and third falls)

THIRD FALLS ALONG TENANT CREEK

GPS COORDINATES: N43° 20.792'   W74° 11.404'

DISTANCE & CONFIGURATION: 4.6-mile out-and-back

HIKING TIME: 3–4 hours

HIGHLIGHTS: Three unique waterfalls

ELEVATION: 1,054' at trailhead, 1,340' at highest point along the trail

ACCESS: Open 24/7; no fees or permits required

MAPS: National Geographic *Adirondack Park, Lake George/Great Sacandaga* (#743)

FACILITIES: Pit toilet

WHEELCHAIR ACCESS: No

COMMENTS: In 2016 the trail was rerouted to avoid a section of trail that crossed private property. December 1–April 1 the last 1.4 miles of Hope Falls Road is closed. To access the trail during these months, park in the pulloff area near the barrier gate and hike Hope Falls Road roughly 1 mile to the new trailhead.

CONTACTS: Eastern Adirondack trail information: www.dec.ny.gov/outdoor/9199.html; emergency contact: 518-891-0235

Overview

Reaching the first of these three beautiful and distinct waterfalls is relatively easy. Its cascading waters over exposed rock faces are impressive and sure to please. Finding the second and third falls requires a bit of bushwhacking along a maze of paths, but the two serene and Zen-like waterfalls are excellent compensation.

Route Details

The trail, marked with yellow trail markers, begins on the western edge of the parking area and climbs slightly northeast to the trail register. From here until the intersection with the old trail at Tenant Creek, 0.8 mile ahead, the path winds around the northeastern contours of Rand Mountain. It adds roughly 0.25 mile of length, 200 feet of climb, and 100 feet of descent to the trail than the previous route, but it's not particularly challenging and makes reaching the first falls just a touch more rewarding. Roughly halfway along the way to the old trail, pass a giant boulder with hemlock growing atop it. The boulder and long sinuous roots of the hemlock are unmistakable and a great landmark to and from the falls. Shortly after passing the boulder, the climbing ends, and you follow a brief flat section and then begin the descent to Tenant Creek. After a looping switchback, rock-hop across a feeder brook and follow this tributary northward to intersect the old trail that wends along Tenant Creek. By now, the roar of the falls is distinct and draws you forward through a coppice of hemlocks to the falls. You will likely leave the trail to scrabble among the myriad paths that weave down to the base of the falls.

Tumbling over a sloping rock face, water falls 40 feet into a large basin at the foot of the falls. Tall hemlocks frame the pool, and numerous boulders along its rocky shore provide places to stop and contemplate the scene. The marked portion of trail ends at the top of the falls, and this is likely as far as many visitors come because the trail—or more accurately, path—is less distinct and practically disappears on occasion as it winds upstream. However, it's hardly a problem, as your

Tenant Creek Falls

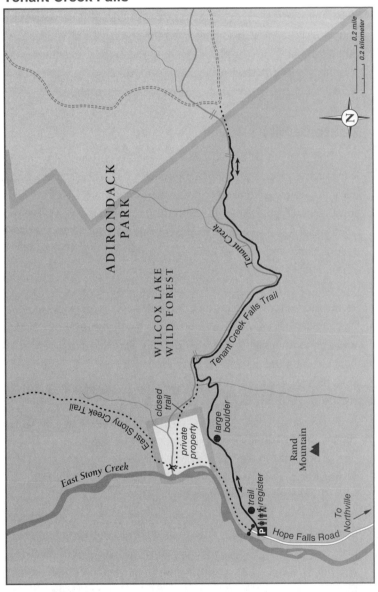

destination is along this creek. If you follow it upstream and keep it on your left, you will find the second and third falls.

Scramble back up to the top of the falls, and begin to pick your way along the creekbank. The transition from trail to multiple paths is at its worst at this point, so stay close to the creek and you will eventually find the trail again. Though it is not difficult, you will have to be nimble to pick your way through the rocks and tangle of roots. The creek forms a small bulge, or horseshoe, around 1.4 miles, after which the flow levels off and the banks become grassy. Around 1.5 miles you will cross a tiny stream, and then the trail climbs slightly uphill away from the creek. The trail follows an elevated ridge briefly and then descends to the creek again. After crossing and recrossing a tiny branch of the creek, you come out on a ledge across from the second falls, which cascade into a broad pool before you. I noticed many salamanders in the pool around the remains of crayfish.

The third falls is a few hundred yards upstream, with the best view from a sloped boulder next to the trail. Both falls are small, but the sheer rock ledges and encroaching forest make each feel wild and isolated. The pools at the bases are deep and enclosed, making excellent spots to take a swim. The roaring of the falls in their mini

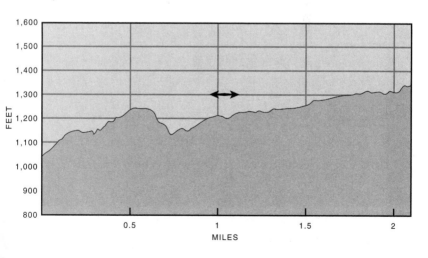

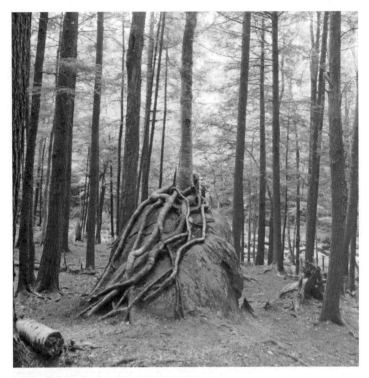

TREE GROWING ATOP ROCK NEAR FIRST FALLS

amphitheaters resonates deeply and drowns out the sounds of the surrounding forest. It is very easy to be drawn in and enchanted by these serene and wild places, so plan to spend some extra time to enjoy the solitude.

Directions

From the intersection of County Road 6/Benson Road and NY 30 in Northville, head north along NY 30. In 0.8 mile, after crossing the Sacandaga River, turn right onto CR 15/Old Northville Road. Continue 1.4 miles, and turn left onto Hope Falls Road/CR 7 (dirt road). Follow the road past several designated primitive campsites to the parking area at 7 miles.

Hadley Mountain

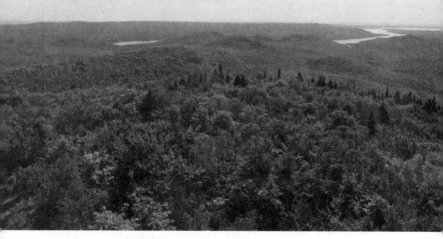

SCENERY: ★ ★ ★ ★ ★
TRAIL CONDITION: ★ ★ ★ ★
CHILDREN: ★ ★ ★ ★
DIFFICULTY: ★ ★ ★
SOLITUDE: ★

VISTA FROM THE SUMMIT OF HADLEY MOUNTAIN

GPS COORDINATES: N43° 22.421'   W73° 57.033'

DISTANCE & CONFIGURATION: 3.6-mile out-and-back

HIKING TIME: 2–3 hours

HIGHLIGHTS: Panoramic views, accessible fire tower

ELEVATION: 1,144' at trailhead, 2,675' at highest point

ACCESS: Open 24/7; no fees or permits required

MAPS: National Geographic *Adirondack Park, Lake George/Great Sacandaga* (#743)

FACILITIES: None

WHEELCHAIR ACCESS: No

CONTACTS: Eastern Adirondack trail information: www.dec.ny.gov/outdoor/9199.html; emergency contact: 518-891-0235

Hadley Mountain

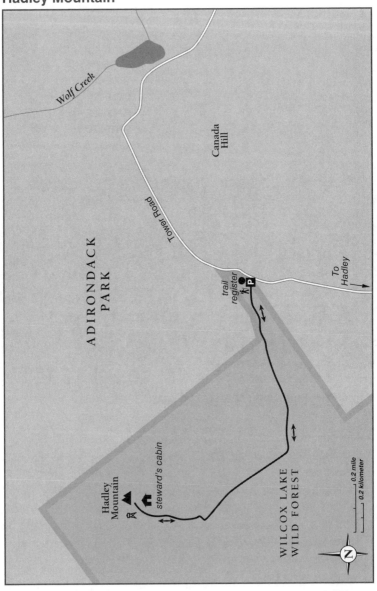

Overview

A short and steady climb to the top of this 2,680-foot bald summit provides great views of the southern Adirondacks. With a climbable fire tower; summertime summit steward; and broad, open mountaintop ideal for a picnic, Hadley Mountain is a great choice for family outings.

Route Details

The trailhead parking area accommodates dozens of vehicles, but the trail's popularity means that you will likely have to park on the side of the dirt access road. The trailhead is clearly marked with a painted Department of Environmental Conservation (DEC) sign, as well as a historical marker detailing the story of the fire tower. Several fires at the opening of the 20th century swept the area, and most of the forest, including the topsoil, was burned off. A wooden tower was erected in 1916, according to a placard, but other sources date it to 1917. After it blew over in severe winds, a steel tower with guylines took its place in 1920. Because the risk of forest fires in the Adirondacks is generally negligible, the use of fire towers for fire suppression has given way to aerial observation; consequently, the tower, cabin, and

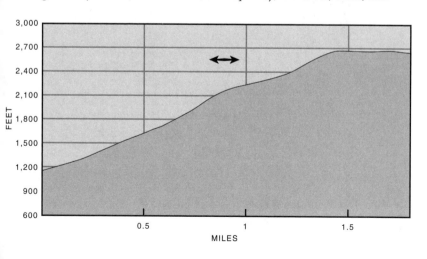

trail fell into disrepair. However, within the past couple of decades, the Hadley Mountain Fire Tower Committee has restored the tower, cabin, and trail, and the old observer's cabin is now manned daily from the Fourth of July until Labor Day by a tower steward. According to the DEC Unit Management Plan, the steward is also available on weekends through Columbus Day.

The beginning of the trail is surrounded by a thick stand of hemlocks that continues to provide shade up to the trail register, where the evergreens give way to a mainly beech and birch forest that is thick with saplings and shades the trail for most of the climb. The trail, marked by red DEC markers, begins to ascend immediately and continues steadily uphill for nearly 1 mile, where it levels off for a while before the final climb to the summit. Over this first section, large rocks and cobbles are strewn across many portions, while other parts proceed up bare bedrock. Chances are that you will need to step off the trail frequently, as many hikers will be either ascending or descending. The trail is so clear that directions are hardly needed.

Upon reaching the ridgeline, views to the southeast glimpsed through the canopy hint at the truly panoramic views that await you shortly ahead. Along the ridgeline, the flora is mostly scrubby trees or saplings, and the trail is largely clear of the rocks and cobbles that previously covered the path. You will pass through a small notch in the bedrock, followed by a sharp turn left before the last climb to the summit. The mountaintop is almost entirely exposed bedrock with many places to sit and enjoy the views. In fact, when I reached the summit, there were more than a dozen families or groups, with ample room for people to spread out to enjoy an afternoon picnic. Panoramic views in all directions are available, and you can see even farther into the surrounding country if you climb the fire tower. To the southwest, you can see Great Sacandaga Lake; to the north, some of the famous High Peaks; to the south, glimpses of the Catskills; and to the east, the foothills surrounding Lake George and even the Green Mountains of Vermont or the Berkshires in Massachusetts. A steady breeze helps to keep the infamous black

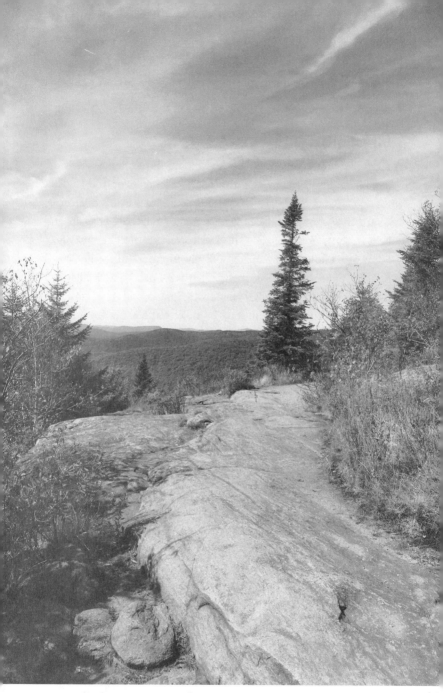

NEAR THE SUMMIT OF HADLEY MOUNTAIN

flies at bay, and with the spectacular views, it is clear why this is a popular picnic spot for families.

Directions

From the intersection of NY 9N/West Maple Street and Main Street in Corinth, head 5.1 miles north on NY 9N, crossing the Hudson River in Hadley, and turn left onto School Street in Lake Luzerne. Continue west onto Bridge Street. Cross the Hudson River again, and keep left onto County Road 4/Rockwell Street. Turn right onto CR 1/ Stony Creek Road, approximately 0.5 mile from your turn onto School Street. Head north on CR 1, and veer left at 3.1 miles onto Hadley Hill Road. Continue along Hadley Hill Road 4.3 miles, and turn right onto Tower Road (dirt road). Continue 1.4 miles north along Tower Road; the trailhead parking area is on the left.

THE FIRE TOWER ATOP HADLEY MOUNTAIN

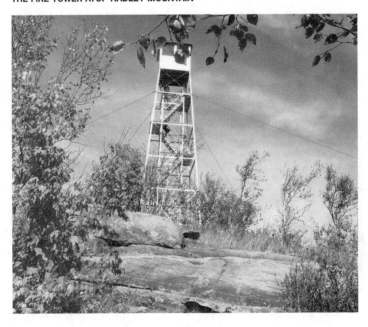

Crane Mountain

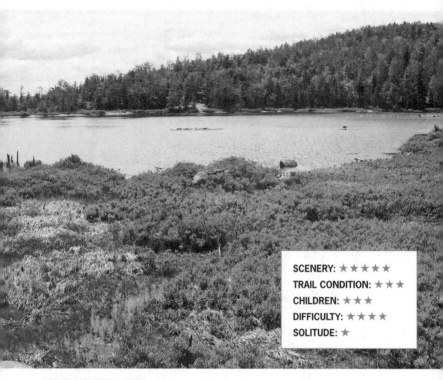

SCENERY: ★ ★ ★ ★ ★
TRAIL CONDITION: ★ ★ ★
CHILDREN: ★ ★ ★
DIFFICULTY: ★ ★ ★ ★
SOLITUDE: ★

CRANE MOUNTAIN POND

GPS COORDINATES: N43° 32.224'   W73° 58.120'

DISTANCE & CONFIGURATION: 4.6-mile loop

HIKING TIME: 5–6 hours

HIGHLIGHTS: Panoramic view, bald summit, pristine pond

ELEVATION: 2,078' at trailhead, 3,254' at highest point

ACCESS: Open 24/7; no fees or permits required

MAPS: National Geographic *Adirondack Park, Lake George/Great Sacandaga* (#743)

FACILITIES: None

WHEELCHAIR ACCESS: No

CONTACTS: Eastern Adirondack trail information: www.dec.ny.gov/outdoor/9199.html; emergency contact: 518-891-0235

Crane Mountain

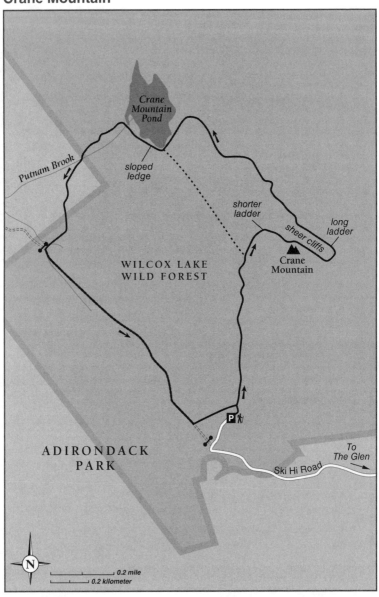

Overview

Crane Mountain is one of the most popular hikes in the southern Adirondacks: with its spectacular views and beautiful mountain pond, it is easy to see why. The climbing is steep, the descent bone-jarring, and the trail varied. It is a wonderful hike, but don't expect privacy, as dozens of groups visit the peak each day.

Route Details

After the long, steep drive up the mountain along Ski Hi Road, you might begin to wonder how much climbing is left. The short answer is: plenty. The trail climbs more than 1,100 feet in less than 0.8 mile. The climb is nearly vertical in sections, and you will have to use both hands in many places. Though it's certainly within the grasp of most hikers and many children, those with bad joints or balance won't find the climb or descent very enjoyable.

Head to the north end of the parking area, where you'll find the trail register a short distance up the trail on your left. Keep right at the fork (to your left is the return leg), and begin climbing among mixed hardwoods. Approximately 0.25 mile in, the vertical climb begins, and you have to pick your way over rough rocks and boulders.

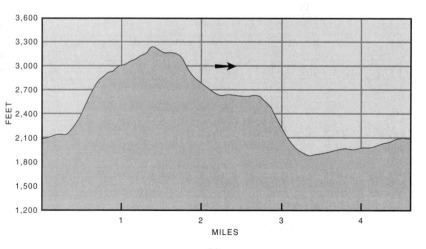

Because of the popularity of the trail, you will likely encounter other hikers along your way. There are many places to step off the trail to let others pass, and many of them are outlooks with outstanding views. At approximately 0.5 mile, the trail swings to the right, and you come out onto an open portion of ledge. Looking straight up the ledge, you will see a rock cairn that indicates where you pick up the trail again. At 0.7 mile, you come to a T; to your left is Crane Mountain Pond, while the right leg is the Crane Mountain summit. Head right toward the summit. The trail leads down, over a small hillock ahead, and then down again to the base of another vertical climb. At 0.8 mile, you come to the first of two wooden ladders that assist hikers over impassable vertical sections. After you climb the short ladder, the trail levels off briefly as it winds through stunted evergreens along the base of the summit's cliff. Chances are that you will see or, at the very least, hear other hikers who are sitting at the mountaintop. After heading east briefly, the trail switchbacks north, and you come to some steeper sections before the summit. A much longer ladder at 1.2 miles signals that the climb is nearly over. Upon reaching the summit at 1.4 miles, you will see numerous open sections along the cliff's edge. Hikers congregate here to enjoy the views and rest after the steep climb. There are plenty of places to rest, so if a section is occupied by another group, continue along the trail, and you will surely find a spot to yourself.

Along the peak, the trail weaves in and out of evergreens to the various lookouts along the cliff's edge. Many of these lookouts are visible from previous points, so you might want to leave someone behind to take a dramatic picture.

The climb down to Crane Mountain Pond is very steep and slippery and has the added hazard of many blown-down pines across the trail. Their whorls of broken branches make a veritable barricade of sharp stakes, so take your time making your way along this descent. The trail begins to level off when you reach a hardwood forest dominated by birches and maples. At 2.3 miles, you will come to a fork in the trail; straight ahead is a short path to an exposed boulder that

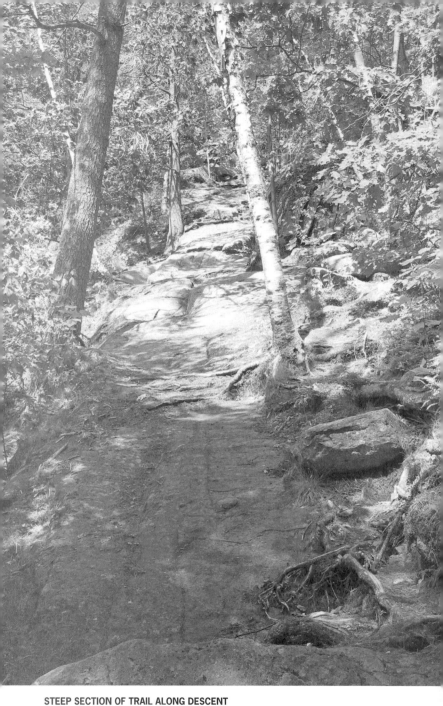

STEEP SECTION OF TRAIL ALONG DESCENT

sits above a wetland on Crane Mountain Pond's southeastern shore. From the fork, the main trail heads to your left and, after a brief foray into the woods, descends to the pond's shore. A fallen tree hides the trail along the shore, but undoubtedly you will have walked to the shore's edge to admire the view. Directly across a tiny bay in the pond is a sloping ledge that gradually enters the water. Hikers also congregate here, as it is popular for swimming. To reach this ledge, continue left along the shore through a small wet area and then though a dense coppice of cedars. Dragonflies will likely dive-bomb you through this section and as you step out onto the ledge. The spur back to the fork, at 0.7 mile, is near this sloped ledge. You can head back along it and then down the initial ascent to the parking area, if you choose not to follow the rest of the trail.

The trail continues to wind along the pond's shore and, after passing a small rocky bay on your right, crosses Putnam Brook. An arrow indicates that the trail continues left, but no mileage or details are given. The footpaths that head off in other directions are angler's paths or bushwhacks. Head west along the main trail, recross Putnam Brook, and come out onto a large, open portion of bedrock. There is no indication as to where the trail picks up again across this open rock face, but if you stick to the northern edge, next to Putnam Brook, you will find it. The trail begins to descend steeply again; be careful and take plenty of time along this stretch, as it is steeper—if you can believe it—than the ascent. The trail is very rocky, and you will likely need to crab-walk or scoot down several sections. Impressive views open up all over to the southwest, but keeping your eyes on the trail should be your main concern. The true path is often hard to discern because you traverse long sections of ledge or hop exclusively from boulder to boulder, both of which mask the footprints of previous hikers. Don't worry though; red Department of Environmental Conservation disks are clearly visible on the many maple trees that shade the trail. After 0.5 mile of descent, the trail levels off, and you will notice a small wetland to your left, around 3.2 miles. Shortly after, cross over the stream that flows out of this wetland along a natural bridge. To either side of the bridge, you will see deep holes. Venturing to the rims of these holes reveals a water-carved cave underneath the bridge. Shortly after crossing, you descend to a feeder stream of Putnam Brook, as well as an intersection with the overgrown Crane Mountain Road. To your right, the road crosses the stream and enters private property, while to your left is a vehicle barrier and the return trip to the parking area. The abandoned road climbs steadily but gently through a mixed hardwood forest back to the parking area. The last mile of the hike is easygoing and free of obstructions, a welcome break from the more difficult ascent and descent. At 4.3 miles, you come to a fork where the road continues straight ahead and a trail heads left. The trail leads to the register and north end of the parking lot. The road intersects Ski Hi Road a few hundred feet south of the parking area.

Directions

From the intersection of NY 28 and NY 8 in Wevertown, head 1.5 miles southwest on NY 8. Turn left onto South Johnsburg Road, and go 6.8 miles. In the hamlet of Thurman, turn right onto County Road 72/Garnet Lake Road. Proceed 1.2 miles, and turn right onto Ski Hi Road. Ski Hi Road is a steep, rough dirt road, but it is maintained and drivable by most cars. Follow Ski Hi Road 1.8 miles, and bear right at the vehicle barrier. The road terminates at the parking area 0.1 mile past the barrier.

West-Central (Hikes 8–14)

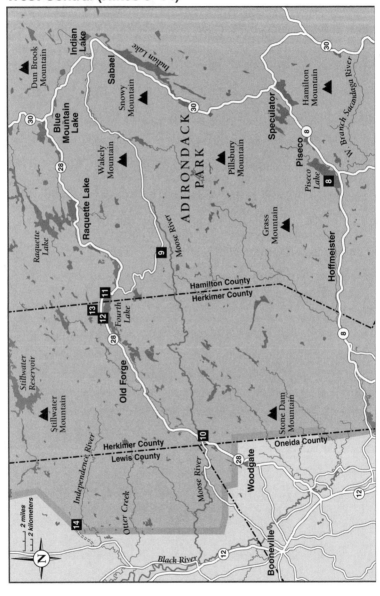

West-Central

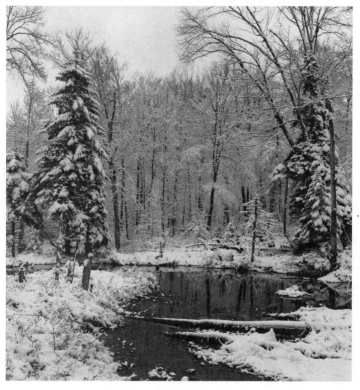

SEASONAL STREAM ON THE WAY TO WOODHULL LAKE *(Trail 10, Bear and Woodhull Lakes, page 80)*

Panther Mountain and Echo Cliffs

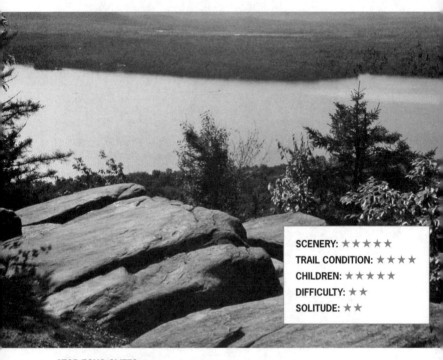

SCENERY: ★ ★ ★ ★ ★
TRAIL CONDITION: ★ ★ ★ ★
CHILDREN: ★ ★ ★ ★ ★
DIFFICULTY: ★ ★
SOLITUDE: ★ ★

ATOP ECHO CLIFFS

GPS COORDINATES: N43° 24.689'   W74° 33.468'

DISTANCE & CONFIGURATION: 1.4-mile out-and-back

HIKING TIME: 1.5 hours

HIGHLIGHTS: Panoramic views

ELEVATION: 1,736' at trailhead, 2,420' at highest point

ACCESS: Open 24/7; no fees or permits required

MAPS: National Geographic *Adirondack Park, Northville/Raquette Lake* (#744)

FACILITIES: None

WHEELCHAIR ACCESS: No

CONTACTS: Central and Southern Adirondack trail information: www.dec.ny.gov/outdoor /9200.html; emergency contact: 518-891-0235

Overview

Definitely the shortest trail described in this book, Panther Mountain and Echo Cliffs are not short on scenery. With less than a mile to the scenic lookout, hikers are quickly rewarded with panoramic views of Piseco Lake. The scenic vista, combined with some stunning cliffs beside the trail, makes it an excellent excursion in one short package. Its popularity in the summer attests to its beauty, so plan on going in the off-season or early morning hours to avoid the crowds.

Route Details

Parking for the Panther Mountain and Echo Cliffs Trail is on the eastern side of County Road 24, just south of the entrance to Little Sand Point Campground. Piseco Lake actually has three campgrounds along its shores; I recommend *Best Tent Camping: New York State* for further descriptions of the campgrounds. Located on the boundary between the west-central and southern regions and fairly close to the central region, Piseco Lake makes a great base camp from which to explore the Adirondack foothills.

Though the trail is often described as Panther Mountain, your actual destination is the ledge along Echo Cliffs. The ledge is 2,420 feet in elevation, 300 feet less than the Panther Mountain summit. The mountain apparently got its name from the abundance of mountain lions, or panthers, in the area in the early 1800s. The town board of Arietta consequently offered a bounty of $20 to purge the area of panthers in 1837. Also known as cougars, the large predators have been absent from New York and the Adirondacks since the 1800s. Rumors abound regarding recent sightings throughout the Adirondacks, and the rumor mill has gone so far as to claim that the Department of Environmental Conservation (DEC) is releasing cougars to curtail the deer population. The rumors have spread wildly through online chat rooms and even sprouted YouTube videos suggesting a conspiracy. The DEC has refuted the claims numerous times and even created a Web page to clarify the issue. The official stance is that

Panther Mountain and Echo Cliffs

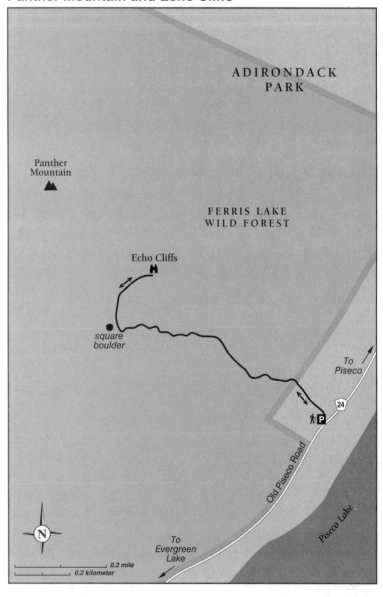

a self-sustaining population of cougars does not exist in New York, that sightings are almost always cases of mistaken identity, and that the extremely rare actual cougars are escapees or releases from private owners.

The parking area is a long pulloff that is about 50 yards long and could easily accommodate dozens of vehicles. A DEC trail sign with a blue disk marks the trailhead on the opposite side of the road.

This trail is ideal for novice hikers, children, or simply a quick climb for a scenic view. Well worn and clearly marked, the path is easy to follow. The trail, marked with blue disks, is obviously popular; heavy use has turned the path into a wide swath along the forest floor. Under the dense canopy of birch, maple, and beech trees, the trail is mostly level as you head generally northwest, but it gradually becomes steeper after you pass through a jumble of angular boulders and begin to head west.

Approximately 0.6 mile in, you pass a large square boulder on your left. After the square boulder, the trail turns north, and you soon pass under sheer rock walls to your left. The trail is much steeper along this section, but the climb is brief, and after you pick your way up the roots of a hemlock tree that grows on the right side

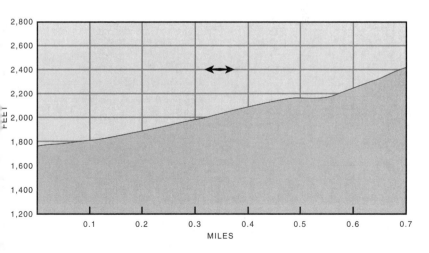

of the trail, you are rewarded with views of Piseco Lake. The lookout is the top of Echo Cliffs, and while the summit of Panther Mountain is behind you to the northwest, no clear path leads to it. The long, exposed outcrop provides a panoramic view of most of Piseco Lake, including Higgins Bay and Spy Lake to the east and directly across the lake, as well as portions of Irondequoit Bay, Big Bay, and the Piseco outlet to the south.

Directions

FROM THE WEST   From the intersection of NY 8 and NY 365 in Cold Brook, head 19.4 miles east on NY 8, and turn left onto County Road 24/Old Piseco Road. Continue 2.6 miles, and look for the pull-off on your right. If you reach Little Sand Point Campground, you are 0.5 mile too far north.

FROM THE EAST   From the intersection of NY 8 and NY 30 in Speculator, head 8.8 miles west on NY 8, and turn right onto CR 24/Old Piseco Road. Follow Old Piseco Road around the northern tip of Piseco Lake, and look for the parking area on your left, 0.5 mile south of Little Sand Point Campground, 5.4 miles along CR 24/Old Piseco Road.

9   # Mitchell Ponds

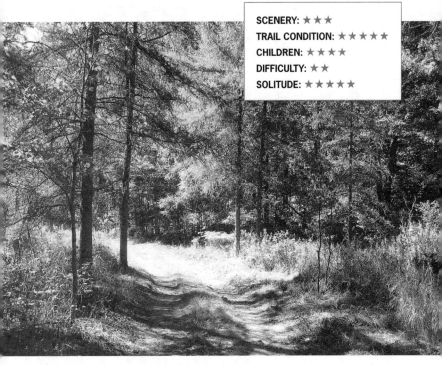

ACCESS ROAD ALONG TRAIL TO MITCHELL PONDS

GPS COORDINATES: N43° 40.589'   W74° 42.490'

DISTANCE & CONFIGURATION: 5.6-mile out-and-back

HIKING TIME: 2–3 hours

HIGHLIGHTS: Lakeside hiking, beaver dam

ELEVATION: 1,839' at trailhead, with no significant rise

ACCESS: Open 24/7; no fees or permits required

MAPS: National Geographic *Adirondack Park, Old Forge/Oswegatchie* (#745); National Geographic *Adirondack Park, Northville/Raquette Lake* (#744)

FACILITIES: None

WHEELCHAIR ACCESS: No

CONTACTS: Moose River Plains Wild Forest: www.dec.ny.gov/lands/53596.html; Central and Southern Adirondack trail information: www.dec.ny.gov/outdoor/9200.html; emergency contact: 518-891-0235

Mitchell Ponds

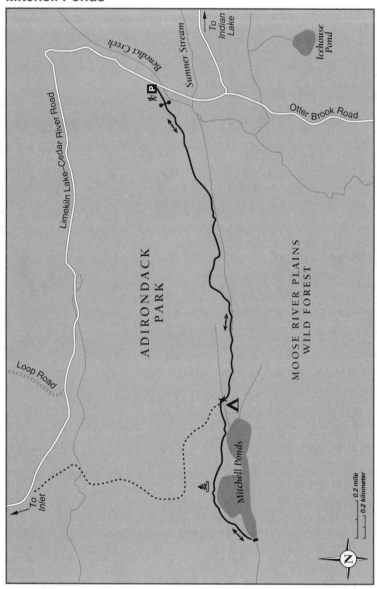

Overview

Nestled in the middle of the Moose River Plains Wild Forest, the trail to Mitchell Ponds is an easy stroll along an old logging road, followed by a quick jaunt along the lake. The trail follows mostly level ground and is easy to follow, so expect to make good time. Trail conditions also make it a great introduction to hiking.

Route Details

To reach Mitchell Ponds, you have to enter the Moose River Plains Wild Forest. Purchased in 1963 from the Gould Paper Company, the 50,000-acre block is bisected by a network of rough roads and myriad roadside campsites—more than 170 mostly primitive sites. The roads are gravelly and filled with potholes and other hazards characteristic of lightly maintained backwoods roads, so a four-wheel-drive, high-clearance vehicle is recommended. Registration booths are at the entrances to the area, and the whole road system is open to vehicles from Memorial Day to the end of hunting season. It is a popular destination during hunting season, and you might think that more vehicles are in the recreation area than on the main roads.

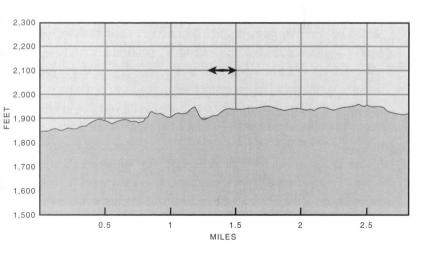

The parking area is essentially an access road, but there is room for a handful of vehicles on either side of the road. The trail, marked with yellow disks, is a continuation of this access road and heads nearly due west. After a few hundred feet, you pass a barrier gate. The trail is mostly level, and because it is an old access road, you can easily walk two abreast. The trail is free from obstructions, so you can easily observe the surrounding landscape as you make good time along the road. At 1.4 miles, you will see a small stream and wetland on the left, though most of the trip is through dense woods.

At 1.8 miles, you reach a clearing and a fork in the trail. Straight ahead is a designated campsite on the eastern tip of Mitchell Ponds. It has a picnic table and beautiful views of the water, making it an ideal stopping point even if you don't plan to camp.

Back at the intersection, the trail continues to your right through a very wet section and over a deteriorating bridge. Just on the other side of the bridge is a second intersection on your left. Straight ahead is the trail that leads to the north access point on Limekiln Lake–Cedar River Road, while the trail along the shores of Mitchell Ponds is on your left. From this point on, the path is no longer a wide forest road but a typical Adirondack foot trail. It weaves along Mitchell Ponds' northern shore, providing views and a tranquil setting. At 2.2 miles, you reach an old fire pit in the midst of the trail and an old sign reminding you of the carry-in, carry-out policy that is in place for the entire Adirondack Park. Past the fire pit, the trail becomes more rugged, narrower, and a little harder to make out, but there is nothing that exceeds the skills of even novice hikers.

Shortly after the fire pit, the trail swings southwest as it weaves its way to the western tip of the ponds. A jumble of boulders fills the steep hillside to your right, forming many small caves and crevices. At 2.8 miles, you reach this tip and the end of the trail, where a beaver dam blocks the outflow of the pond. You can get a few views back on the ponds from the large rocks, but crossing the outlet would probably be wet and difficult. Return the way you came for a round-trip of 5.6 miles.

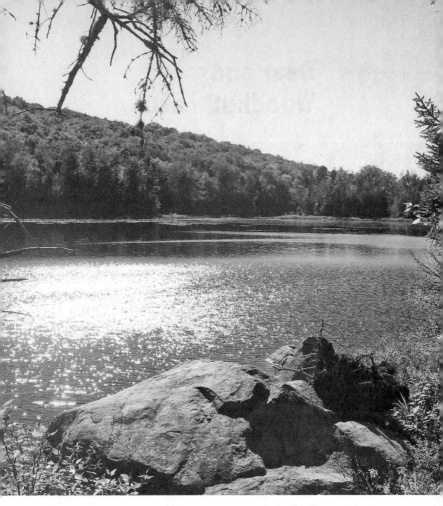

MITCHELL PONDS

Directions

From NY 28 in Inlet, 0.8 mile east of the intersection of NY 28 and South Shore Road in Inlet and 9.8 miles west of the intersection of Sagamore Road and NY 28 in Raquette Lake, head southwest on Limekiln Lake Road/County Road 14. Continue 1.9 miles on Limekiln Lake Road to the registration booth. From the registration booth, follow Limekiln Lake–Cedar River Road east and south 8.1 miles. The parking area is on your right.

Bear and Woodhull Lakes

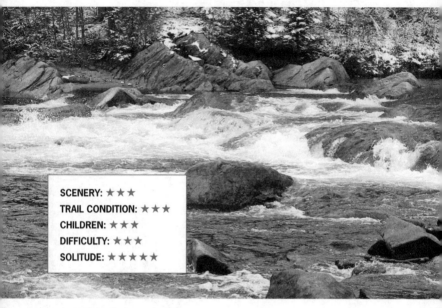

SCENERY: ★ ★ ★
TRAIL CONDITION: ★ ★ ★
CHILDREN: ★ ★ ★
DIFFICULTY: ★ ★ ★
SOLITUDE: ★ ★ ★ ★ ★

REMSEN FALLS

GPS COORDINATES: N43° 36.749'   W75° 05.429'

DISTANCE & CONFIGURATION: 10.2-mile loop, 1.2-mile out-and-back side trip

HIKING TIME: 5–7 hours

HIGHLIGHTS: Lakeside hiking, waterfall

ELEVATION: 1,547' at trailhead, 2,003' at highest point

ACCESS: Open 24/7; no fees or permits required

MAPS: National Geographic *Adirondack Park, Old Forge/Oswegatchie* (#745)

FACILITIES: None

WHEELCHAIR ACCESS: Yes, along Remsen Falls side trip

COMMENTS: A newly constructed lean-to is available at Bear Lake, in addition to the popular lean-to at Woodhull Lake.

CONTACTS: Central and Southern Adirondack trail information: www.dec.ny.gov/outdoor /9200.html; Black River Wild Forest: www.dec.ny.gov/lands/75310.html; emergency contact: 518-891-0235

Overview

More than half of the loop to Bear and Woodhull Lakes includes gravel and dirt access roads, but these roads are closed to traffic or lightly traveled. The trail portions are truly excellent and include two lakes, a pond, and seasonal streams to hike beside. A side trip to Remsen Falls is easily accessible along the loop as well. The Remsen Falls side trip is wheelchair accessible, with a special parking area located closer to the falls.

Route Details

The trail network in the Woodhull Lake area is bisected by a gravel road that provides access to several designated roadside campsites as well as the wheelchair-accessible Remsen Falls picnic and camping area. If camping is part of your agenda, you may want to consider the roadside sites or backpack to the lean-to and designated sites by Woodhull Lake. Camping in other areas is permitted as long as you follow the basic backcountry camping guidelines laid out by the Department of Environmental Conservation (DEC). The best parking is available in the McKeever parking area at the end of McKeever Spur Road. Hiking counterclockwise around the loop brings you into the wilderness soonest and leaves the easier roadside hiking for the return trip.

From the parking area, head southeast past the barrier gate along the gravel road. The road climbs gently but is free of obstruction, so you quickly cover the first 0.7 mile and reach the first designated campsite. You pass a second campsite within a couple hundred feet, a bridge at 0.8 mile, and yet another campsite at 1.1 miles. You reach the beginning of the foot trail on your right at 1.3 miles. The trail sign indicates that to your right are Bear Lake, 1.7 miles, and Bear Creek parking area, 8.8 miles. Continuing straight, you reach Remsen Falls in 2.4 miles, Woodhull Mountain in 6.9 miles, and Woodhull Lean-To in 4.6 miles. This intersection is immediately before another bridge.

Head south (right) on the blue-marked trail toward Bear Lake. The trail immediately traverses a flat, wet section that could easily

Bear and Woodhull Lakes

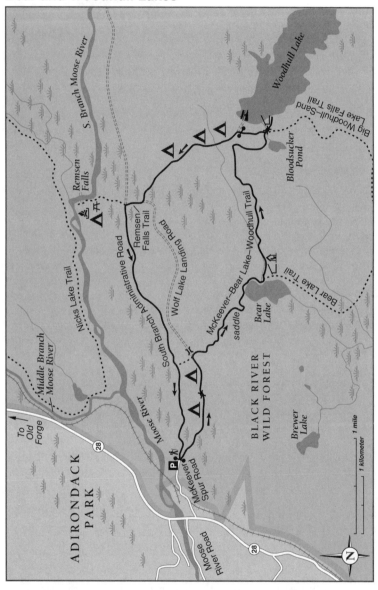

swallow a boot or two. The trail climbs more than 300 feet over the next 0.5 mile through the familiar birch, beech, and maple forest of the western Adirondacks. You reach the crest of your climb at 1.9 miles in a saddle between two hills, where glimpses of Bear Lake are heavily obscured by the forest canopy but promise a picturesque destination. As you weave your way down the next 0.5 mile to the lake, steep ledges become exposed on your left. More than 40 feet high in sections, the ledges reinforce the rugged wilderness feel that hikers so frequently seek along the myriad trails of the Adirondacks. Depending on the season and water level, you might be privy to a tiny waterfall cascading along these ledges around 2.3 miles. Certainly not a frothing cascade, the rivulet breaks through a cleft in the ledge and is seasonal. The trail's descent ends abruptly on the shores of Bear Lake, which is admirably framed before you by a large black cherry tree. A little farther along the trail is an abandoned fire ring, where more exceptional views of the lake await.

The trail winds its way along the northern and then eastern shore of Bear Lake for the next 0.3 mile, where you encounter a feeder stream. After rock-hopping across the stream, you will find a trail intersection on the opposite shore. Straight along the blue-marked trail is Bear Lake Trail, 1.9 miles, and the Bear Creek parking

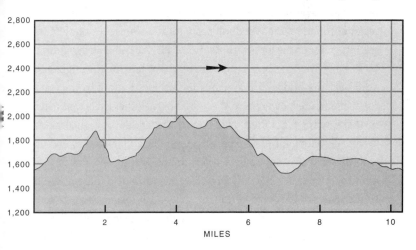

area, 6.9 miles. To your left and marked in yellow are the Woodhull Lean-To, 2.4 miles, and Remsen Falls, 5.2 miles. Continue to your left (east) along the yellow-marked trail.

The trail parallels the stream for the next 0.3 mile as you begin to climb away from Bear Lake. While traversing this section of the trail, I encountered several colors of flagging tape riddled with notes. Because it was hunting season, I first suspected that it was the work of hunters trying to retrace their steps. After a while, the magnitude of the flagging and the consistent spacing showed that it was instead the work of rescue crews trying to find a lost hunter. Every year, hunters and hikers get lost in the woods, and many are not found. Upon returning to civilization, I learned that this case had a happy ending; the hunter was found miles away after spending two cold November nights alone in the woods. Not all are as fortunate, and it is a stark reminder that it is essential to communicate your plans and have regular check-ins.

As you near the crest of your climb, 4.3 miles, the trail swings south. This southern jog of 0.4 mile brings you close to the shores of Bloodsucker Pond, a small pond fed by a stream from Woodhull Lake. When you reach the pond and stream, 4.7 miles, the trail swings east again, and the stream accompanies you as you head east another 0.1 mile to a major trail intersection. To your right is a series of trails that takes you deeper into the Black River Wild Forest as well as to our major destination, the Woodhull Lean-To, at 0.3 mile. To your left are the return leg of the loop with Remsen Falls, 2.5 miles away, and the McKeever parking area, 5.4 miles. To reach the lean-to, turn right and head over the bridge into a giant mire, where the trail to the lean-to, marked in red, diverges to the left from the other trails that delve further into the Black River Wild Forest. The trail down to the lean-to is basically a long mire, so expect to be nimble and inevitably end up with muddy boots anyway. As you near the lean-to, you first notice a pit toilet and, if you're anything like me, can't help but wonder if future routes might avoid long mires that end at toilets. Regardless of your musings on trail routing, you reach the large lean-to on Wood-hull Lake shortly after, 5 miles overall. It has obviously been worked

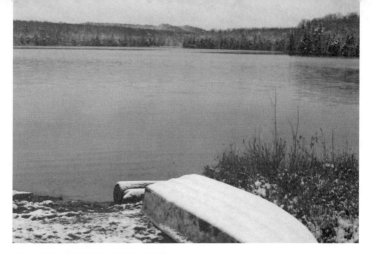

BOAT ON THE SHORE OF BEAR LAKE

on recently and is the equivalent of two lean-tos. Situated within 10 feet of the shore, it has wonderful views and is a great stopping point. But be forewarned, it is a popular destination and, due to its proximity to the road, likely occupied. Return through the mire to the intersection you encountered before the bridge to continue along the loop, 5.2 miles from the start.

Heading north from the intersection, you will follow red snowmobile markers and quickly reach a vehicle barrier gate. The road you intersect continues to the right down to Wolf Lake Landing, but you will head to your left (north) toward Remsen Falls. Pass several campsites as you head north 1.1 miles along the road to the next major intersection. This intersection is just past two closely spaced campsites and is marked by a trail sign. The designated parking area for the wheelchair-access road to Remsen Falls is at this intersection. To the right is Remsen Falls, 0.6 mile, while continuing along the main access road to your left takes you back to the McKeever parking area in 3 miles. Even if you don't plan to take the side trip to Remsen Falls, a more pleasant return leg is along the red-marked trail.

Continue to your right along the wheelchair-access road, marked in red, another 0.1 mile, where you reach another intersection. To your right is Woodhull Mountain, 4.5 miles; straight ahead is Remsen Falls, 0.5 mile; and to your left is the return trip to the McKeever parking area, 3.1 miles.

Side Trip to Remsen Falls

(Mileage along loop does not include this 1.2-mile trip.)

The side trip to Remsen Falls adds 1.2 miles to your total trip, but because it follows wheelchair-accessible paths, this diversion takes little time and effort. Heading almost due north along the wide, flat, and sandy access path, you quickly reach Moose River just above the falls. You can see a lean-to on the opposite shore, and you find a fire pit, picnic table, and designated camping area at the end of the trail. Continue along well-worn paths past the picnic table to get farther downriver to view the falls. When you reach a second picnic table, the falls are clearly visible. Less of a falls and more of a broad rapid, the tumble of water drowns out most surrounding sounds. Another fire pit is located farther downstream if you desire more privacy. Return the way you came to complete the loop.

Back on the main trail, head west along the dirt access road, marked in red. This access road is closed to vehicles, though you might see mountain bikers, as this is a popular biking area. The return trip is mostly level and easygoing and passes without incident. You pass a large culvert at 8 miles, Bear Lake Trail on your left at 8.9 miles, a second culvert at 9.1 miles, and a trail register at 9.8 miles. This second register seems to be used primarily by people visiting the falls or heading straight to the mountain. Head past the barrier gate, where there is a large turnaround, and continue west to the McKeever parking area for a total trip length of 10.2 miles, 11.4 including the side trip.

Directions

From NY 28, turn east onto McKeever Road, 16.2 miles northeast of the intersection of NY 12 and NY 28 in Alder Creek or 10.4 miles southwest of Old Forge. Continue to your right onto McKeever Spur Road at 0.3 mile, past an old railroad station. Continue another 0.4 mile. The parking area is on your right and marked with DEC signs.

Black Bear Mountain

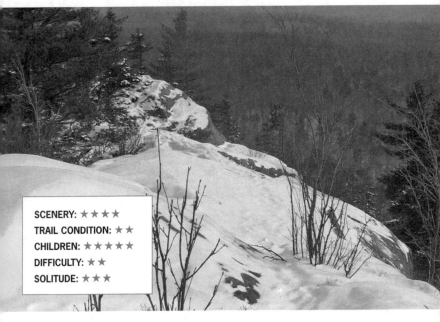

SCENERY: ★ ★ ★ ★
TRAIL CONDITION: ★ ★
CHILDREN: ★ ★ ★ ★ ★
DIFFICULTY: ★ ★
SOLITUDE: ★ ★ ★

NEAR BLACK BEAR PEAK

GPS COORDINATES: N43° 45.808'   W74° 47.572'

DISTANCE & CONFIGURATION: 4.9-mile loop

HIKING TIME: 3 hours

HIGHLIGHTS: Bald mountain, scenic views

ELEVATION: 1,751' at trailhead, 2,432' at highest point

ACCESS: Open 24/7; no fees or permits required

MAPS: National Geographic *Adirondack Park, Old Forge/Oswegatchie* (#745); National Geographic *Adirondack Park, Northville/Raquette Lake* (#744)

FACILITIES: None

WHEELCHAIR ACCESS: No

COMMENTS: Be aware that the first section of the trail is a multiuse trail and mountain biking is becoming more popular in the region. The trail to the summit is hiking only.

CONTACTS: Moose River Plains Wild Forest: www.dec.ny.gov/lands/53596.html; Central and Southern Adirondack trail information: www.dec.ny.gov/outdoor/9200.html; emergency contact: 518-891-0235

Black Bear Mountain

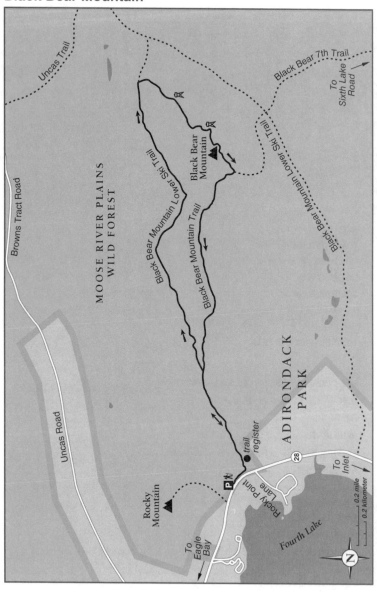

Overview

A popular destination in summer and fall, this tiny peak provides views of the Fulton Chain of Lakes. It is a great choice for children and beginner hikers, but if you wish for solitude, then plan to go during the off-season, especially winter.

Route Details

From the southeast corner of the parking area, head south, paralleling the road. After passing a deteriorating concrete bridge on your left, you will quickly reach a sign indicating the trailhead to your left (east). The trail register is just inside the treeline. The trail—marked in yellow hiking, skiing, and biking disks—heads northeast through mixed hardwoods. Approximately 0.3 mile in, a stream becomes visible on your left. At 0.7 mile you reach the intersection with the return leg of the trip on your right. This trail, also marked in yellow, is a more direct and steeper ascent to the peak, but returning along this trail provides some great views along the descent.

To make the longer and more scenic loop, continue northeast along the left fork (east) through some muddy sections. At approximately 1 mile, you reach a clearing encircled by small firs, with rock

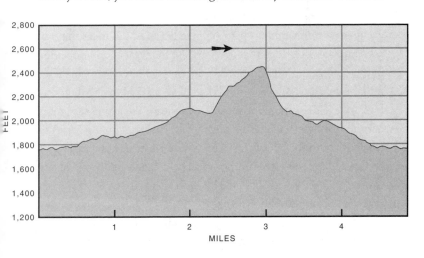

cairns marking the path. Shortly after, you cross a couple of streams over log-and-plank bridges and will soon see the mountain looming off to your right. The grade along the north side of the mountain is relatively flat, and you soon reach another trail intersection at 2.3 miles, just before the halfway point. To your left are Uncas Trail, 0.6 mile, and Uncas Road parking area, 1.5 miles. To your right are the summit, 0.5 mile, and the return to NY 28, 2.6 miles.

The trail begins to climb immediately, and the forest transitions from maple and beech to evergreens fairly quickly. A quarter mile from the intersection, 2.5 miles from the start, you reach an opening in the evergreens and a lookout on your left. From here you have an incredible view of Seventh Lake, part of the Fulton Chain of Lakes.

The Fulton Chain is a series of connected lakes that begins at Old Forge Pond and ends with Eighth Lake. It is a popular destination for a wide variety of boaters and is the beginning of the North Forest Canoe Trail. In fact, First through Fifth Lakes compose an unbroken length of 14 miles. A series of channels separates Old Forge Pond and Sixth through Eighth Lakes from this main expanse. The connection of these lakes was part of steamboat inventor Robert Fulton's vision of an Adirondack Canal. Though the canal was never built, the chain still bears Fulton's name.

Returning to the trail, the path winds in and out of stands of evergreens and over long spans of open ledge. At 2.8 miles the trail runs into a 4-foot ledge that you navigate to reveal another opening in the canopy and yet another lookout on your left. Head northeast into the dense evergreens to find the yellow-marked trail that quickly leads you to the summit about 0.1 mile ahead. The actual summit is hard to distinguish along the mostly flat, bald peak, but a series of small ledges to the left of the trail makes a great spot to dangle your feet and enjoy the view. To the south, you can see portions of the town of Inlet as well as Sixth and Seventh Lakes. To the west, you can make out portions of Fourth Lake.

The trail back to the parking area heads generally west but is now mostly marked with blue trail disks. The descent is steeper than the

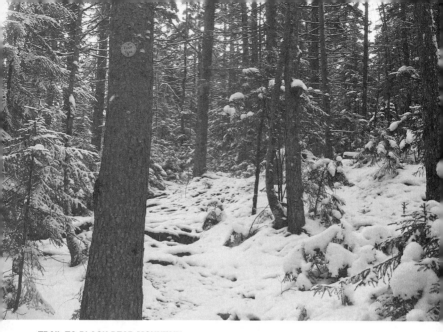

TRAIL TO BLACK BEAR MOUNTAIN

ascent but provides better views of Fourth Lake than any of the look-outs or even the summit. After you weave your way down the many small ledges, some 0.4 mile from the peak, the trail levels off, and you encounter a few more wet areas. At 3.7 miles the blue markers begin to thin, and yellow markers become more prevalent. After a short jog where the trail swings north, the return trail parallels the inbound trail awhile and, after descending along a broad road, you reach the first intersection at 4.2 miles. Hike the remaining 0.7 mile back to NY 28 and the parking area for a total trip length of 4.9 miles.

Directions

Coming from the west, from the junction of County Road 1/Big Moose Road and NY 28 in Eagle Bay, head east on NY 28 and go 1.2 miles. The spacious parking lot is on your left. From the east, from the junction of County Road 1/South Shore Road and NY 28 in Inlet, head north 0.9 mile along NY 28, and look for the parking area on your right. There are two entrances, so if you miss the first in either direction, simply enter the second.

Bubb, Sis, and Moss Lakes

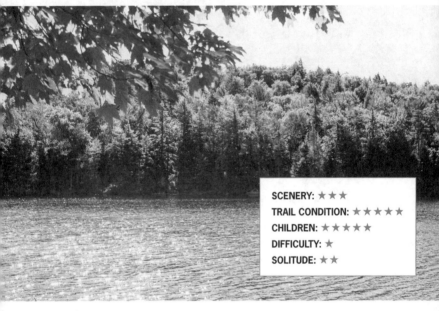

SCENERY: ★ ★ ★
TRAIL CONDITION: ★ ★ ★ ★ ★
CHILDREN: ★ ★ ★ ★ ★
DIFFICULTY: ★
SOLITUDE: ★ ★

BUBB LAKE

GPS COORDINATES: Sis and Bubb parking: N43° 46.001' W74° 50.675'
Moss Lake parking: N43° 47.386' W74° 50.763'

DISTANCE & CONFIGURATION: 7.0-mile balloon

HIKING TIME: 3–4 hours

HIGHLIGHTS: Lakeside hiking

ELEVATION: 1,741' at trailhead, 1,924' at highest point

ACCESS: Open 24/7; no fees or permits required

MAPS: Fulton Chain Map: www.dec.ny.gov/lands/75305.html; National Geographic *Adirondack Park, Old Forge/Oswegatchie* (#745)

FACILITIES: None

WHEELCHAIR ACCESS: Portions of the trail and day area at Moss Lake are accessible.

CONTACTS: Fulton Chain Wild Forest: www.dec.ny.gov/lands/75305.html; Central and Southern Adirondack trail information: www.dec.ny.gov/outdoor/9200.html; emergency contact: 518-891-0235

Overview

These three pristine lakes offer a variety of activities and feature trails with varying levels of accessibility, making this an ideal trip for the entire family. The Moss Lake circuit, with its broad, flat trails and wheelchair-accessible sections, provides an opportunity for the very young—or those no longer interested in hiking rugged trails—to enjoy the beauty of the Adirondacks. On the other hand, the Bubb and Sis Lakes section features rugged trails and remote lakes that are easily combined with the circuit for extended and more invigorating trips.

Route Details

There are a variety of ways to explore these pristine lakes. The Moss Lake circuit has long sections that are wheelchair accessible, and the majority of the trail is flat, broad, and easy to navigate. Two larger parking areas are also available near Moss Lake along Big Moose Road (also known as County Road 1). These parking areas should be used for extended stays, end-to-end hikes, and day use in the Moss Lake area because the Bubb and Sis parking area can realistically accommodate only five to six vehicles, and two of those spaces are designated handicapped parking. You can make it an end-to-end hike if you start at the Bubb and Sis trailhead along NY 28 and get picked up or meet at one of the Moss Lake parking areas along Big Moose Road. The trip described here includes taking a straight route past Bubb and Sis Lakes, then following the circuit around Moss Lake, and finally returning along the straight route between Bubb and Sis Lakes.

The trail, marked with yellow disks, begins in the northwest corner of the small parking area along NY 28. The trail climbs immediately, and after a few dozen yards you reach the trail register. The trail then swings north with a steep incline, and you quickly reach the intersection with the Vista Trail, marked in blue, on your left. Continue straight ahead (northwest), and the trail soon levels off. It is mostly level from this point on, and within 0.5 mile of the start, Bubb Lake comes into view. You encounter a minor fork just before

Bubb, Sis, and Moss Lakes

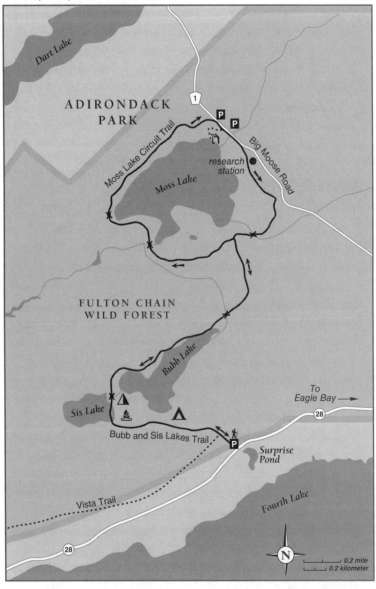

the lakeshore. To the left is the main trail, while straight ahead are an excellent point from which to view the lake and a designated camp-site nestled off to the right of the short path that leads to the lake.

Continuing left (west) along the main trail, you'll cross a small stream as you skirt the southern edge of Bubb Lake. Within min-utes you'll reach a stand of hemlocks along the edge of Sis Lake. In the height of summer, this is a very tranquil area, and the calls of loons can be heard throughout. From this grove of hemlocks, the trail swings north and passes an informal campsite on the left. This site has benches, a fire pit, and an informal path that follows the western edge of Bubb Lake. Just past this site is a boardwalk, 0.8 mile, that crosses the small wetland between the two lakes.

Once on the opposite shore, the trail swings east and follows the northern shore of Bubb Lake. After 0.8 mile you reach the northeastern tip of the lake and encounter yet another heavily used area to the right of the trail. There are several fishing regulation signs, and a bit farther east off the trail is a fire pit. The main trail veers to the left of this heav-ily used area, and at 1.6 miles you cross a small stream over a log-and-plank bridge and notice a wooden dam on the left. The trail becomes broader after this crossing and soon swings north as it heads to the Moss Lake circuit, which you reach at 2.3 miles. To the right is the most

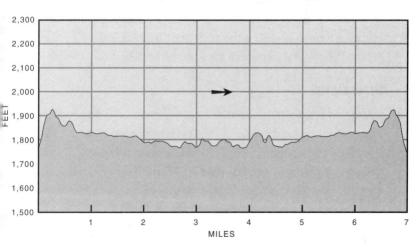

direct route to the parking areas along Big Moose Road and the day-use areas around the lake. Turn left and head clockwise around the circuit.

The trail around Moss Lake is broad and sandy and easily accommodates two or more abreast. It is a popular circuit for groups of walkers, so don't expect much solitude. The lake is hidden from view until you reach a bridge that crosses a stream and wetland that sprawls out to the west. Climb a short hill, and wind your way north along the western edge of the lake. At mile 3.1 cross another log-and-plank bridge, after which the trail swings northeast. As you near the eastern edge of the lake, you pass a road that intersects the trail on the left, 3.7 miles, and head into the day-use area of the lake. Dotting the eastern shore are myriad paths, picnic areas, and designated campsites, as well as an observation deck, that are more easily explored than described. The circuit path bypasses most of these areas and soon reaches the first of two parking areas. At the second parking area is a trail register, campsite register, historical information placard, and map of the circuit and campsites.

Continuing along the main circuit, you'll pass side trails leading to a couple of campsites on your right and then enter an open field with a research station with tall fences off to the left. At 4.3 miles, you pass a side trail to the left that leads to Big Moose Road, followed by a bridge that crosses Moss Lake's main inlet. You soon reach the intersection with the Bubb and Sis Lakes Trail, 4.7 miles. Return the way you came for a total trip of 7 miles.

Directions

SIS AND BUBB LAKES PARKING AREA   From the intersection of Crosby Boulevard and NY 28 in Old Forge, head northeast 7.9 miles along NY 28; the parking area is on the left. From the intersection of County Road 1/Big Moose Road and NY 28 in Eagle Bay, head southwest 1.4 miles along NY 28; the parking area is on your right.

MOSS LAKE PARKING AREA   From NY 28 in Eagle Bay, head north 2.2 miles on CR 1/Big Moose Road; the large parking area is on your left.

13

Cascade Lake

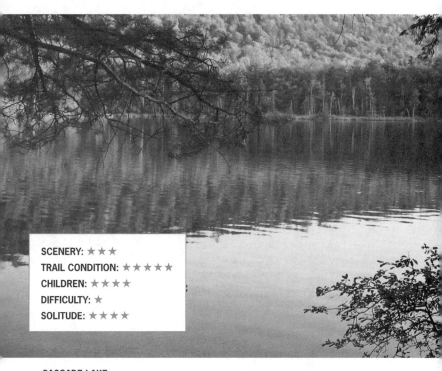

SCENERY: ★ ★ ★
TRAIL CONDITION: ★ ★ ★ ★ ★
CHILDREN: ★ ★ ★ ★
DIFFICULTY: ★
SOLITUDE: ★ ★ ★ ★

CASCADE LAKE

GPS COORDINATES: N43° 46.887'   W74° 49.909'

DISTANCE & CONFIGURATION: 5.9-mile balloon

HIKING TIME: 3–4 hours

HIGHLIGHTS: Lakeside hiking, tall waterfall, historic site

ELEVATION: 1,873' at trailhead, 1,940' at highest point

ACCESS: Open 24/7; no fees or permits required

MAPS: National Geographic *Adirondack Park, Old Forge/Oswegatchie* (#745)

FACILITIES: None

WHEELCHAIR ACCESS: No

CONTACTS: Pigeon Lake Wilderness Area: www.dec.ny.gov/lands/102484.html; Central and Southern Adirondack trail information: www.dec.ny.gov/outdoor/9200.html; emergency contact: 518-891-0235

Cascade Lake

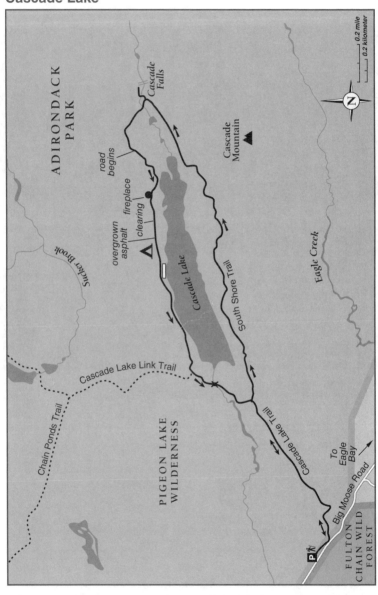

Overview

Not to be confused with Cascade Lake in the High Peaks region, this scenic loop in the town of Inlet offers an excellent trip around the lake and includes a 43-foot waterfall. The roughly 6-mile circuit follows old access roads that are wide enough for two to walk side by side nearly the entire way. Wonderful camping spots are found along the north shore.

Route Details

The trailhead is located in the southeast corner of the spacious parking area along Big Moose Road. A painted map of the Pigeon Lake Wilderness trail system is also located next to the trail register. The trail briefly parallels the road in a southeasterly direction before swinging east under the canopy of pole-size hardwoods. Trail markers switch between yellow cross-country skiing disks and red foot-trail disks. Because most of the trail is along old access roads, it would be hard to lose your way. The roads once led to Camp Cascade, originally a summer camp for Charles E. Snyder that easily could have been considered one of the "Great Camps." It was later sold at a fraction of the asking price to Dr. George Longstaff. Longstaff, already an owner of

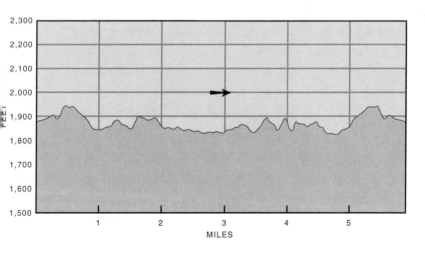

a sailing camp on nearby Moss Lake, transformed the property into an all-girls equestrian camp. When the camp began to falter during World War II, it became coed. The state acquired the property in 1962 and had plans to build a campground, but shortly afterward the state removed the buildings in accordance with the Forever Wild initiative.

About 0.3 mile in, you intersect this old road and begin to head northeast. As it was in the past, the broad road is clearly used by horses in the summer (watch your step) and would make a great skiing trail in the winter. Numerous wet spots dot the road but are easily bypassed along the shoulders. At 1 mile the road intersects the south-shore trail on your right. Though the south-shore trail parallels the lake's southern shore, you will not be able to see the lake until you reach the eastern tip near the waterfall. However, the circuit seems to make the most sense hiked in a counterclockwise direction, so mileage and directions are given accordingly.

The forest matures as you head farther along the trail, and two can walk easily abreast for almost the entire circuit. A few mucky areas sprawl across the trail during the next couple of miles, but overall it is a very pleasant woodland walk. At 2.5 miles you catch your first glimpse of the lake as the forest becomes thicker with evergreens. Roughly 3 miles from the parking area, you come across an open meadow with a stream cutting its way west to Cascade Lake. Head a brief distance east into the surrounding forest, along any of the numerous footpaths, to find the namesake waterfall. The narrow cascade falls 43 feet onto the rocks below before trickling out into the meadow. To the right of the falls is a path that climbs through a narrow passage to the top. The plateau of bedrock at the top is ideal for sitting and enjoying the falls.

Continuing along the loop, the trail quickly reaches a long wet and muddy section. Stay on the path and pick your footing carefully, as the broad marshland will quickly suck the ill-placed foot knee-deep into the muck. As I can attest, you will likely have to wait until you reach the lakeshore, almost 0.5 mile ahead, before you can wash off the black muck. Upon reentering the woods, the trail weaves uphill briefly before joining the north-shore road at 3.3 miles. The north-shore road drops down to the lake at 3.5 miles and skirts it fairly closely for the next mile with views of the water as well as a few remnants of the abandoned girls camp. The first relic is an old stone fireplace and foundation approximately 0.1 mile after reaching the lake. Small hardwood saplings are starting to reclaim this clearing and many of the other sites farther along. The camp stopped operating in the 1950s and was acquired by the state in 1962, so the regenerative growth is a great example of how quickly nature reasserts itself. The

CASCADE FALLS IN THE HEIGHT OF SUMMER

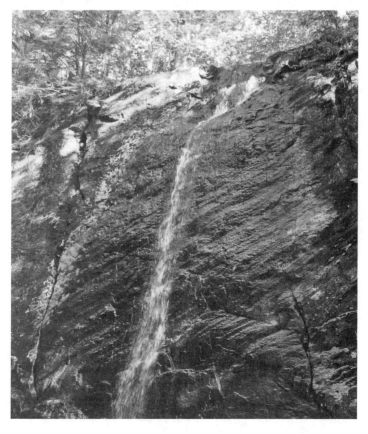

next clearing has a thick carpet of ferns, with dense eastern white pine regeneration that will quickly close in the open space. The most striking reestablishment is at 3.8 miles, where an old tennis court is being broken up and covered by a carpet of grass to the left of the trail. Saplings form a thicket around this formerly impervious surface, and you can tell that it won't be long before roots begin to assist the grasses in breaking up the surface.

Many of these clearings would make great campsites, but the more popular ones, found farther along, have better views of the lake. None of the sites are designated (they're often referred to as informal sites), so Department of Environmental Conservation regulations dictate that you must be 150 feet from both the lake and the trail. One such grassy location is found near the lakeshore a little past the tennis court. Probably the most desirable and likely occupied lakeside campsite is found at 4 miles. An old stone retaining wall holds back the forest on your right, while a heavily shaded lawn sprawls out on your left. The parklike setting is an obvious destination, and its proximity to the road means that weekend campers likely pack in far more than the backcountry camper could. Shortly after, you leave the shores of the lake and reach a fork in the trail. A trail to the right, 4.5 miles from the start, heads to Chain Ponds, Queer Lake, Chub Pond, and the rest of the Pigeon Lake Wilderness. Continue straight ahead (southwest) 0.1 mile to a short steel bridge that crosses the outlet of Cascade Lake. A broad, picturesque wetland sprawls out on your right, and you notice substantial beaver activity in the vicinity. Immediately after, pass by another clearing to the left of the trail and quickly reach the intersection with the south-shore trail. From here, it is another mile back to the parking area.

Directions

From NY 28 in Eagle Bay, head north on County Road 1/Big Moose Road. The spacious parking lot is 1.3 miles on the right.

14

Gleasmans Falls

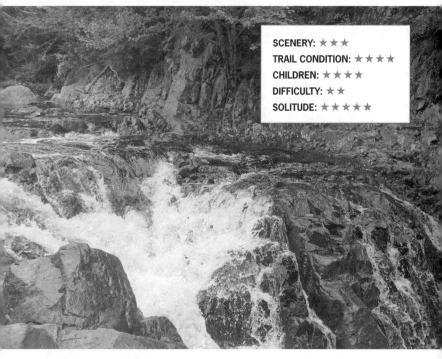

SCENERY: ★ ★ ★
TRAIL CONDITION: ★ ★ ★ ★
CHILDREN: ★ ★ ★ ★
DIFFICULTY: ★ ★
SOLITUDE: ★ ★ ★ ★ ★

TOP OF GLEASMANS FALLS

GPS COORDINATES: N43° 48.490'   W75° 16.589'

DISTANCE & CONFIGURATION: 5.8-mile out-and-back

HIKING TIME: 2–3 hours

HIGHLIGHTS: Beaver dam, series of small waterfalls cascading in a narrow gorge

ELEVATION: 1,290' at trailhead, 1,350' at highest point

ACCESS: Open 24/7; no fees or permits required

MAPS: adirondackstughill.com/maps/BeachMillTrails.pdf; National Geographic *Adirondack Park, Old Forge/Oswegatchie* (#745)

FACILITIES: None

WHEELCHAIR ACCESS: No

CONTACTS: Independence River Wild Forest: www.dec.ny.gov/lands/58192.html; Central and Southern Adirondack trail information: www.dec.ny.gov/outdoor/9200.html; emergency contact: 518-891-0235

Gleasmans Falls

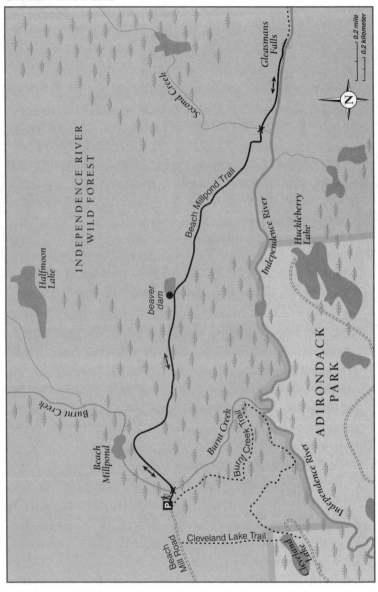

Overview

Situated on the western fringe of the park boundary, this relatively level out-and-back hike is a great trip for hikers who like a little solitude when they arrive at their destination. The falls roar through a narrow gorge, and you can view this torrent from high atop the gorge's sheer walls. Another unique feature is a close-up view of an old beaver dam along the trail.

Route Details

After driving up the long, bumpy road, you will already feel removed from the rest of the world. Indeed, finding the parking area among the unnamed roads will likely be the hardest aspect of this clearly defined trail. You will be following the Beach Millpond Trail, which provides access to a more extensive trail system in the Independence River Wild Forest. From the parking area, you walk down a gravelly path to an open, grassy area with a winding, tannin-laden creek. Burnt Creek is the outflow of the previously dammed Beach Millpond, where a sawmill once produced lumber. You will have to negotiate a few small muddy spots on the way to a recently constructed wooden footbridge. On the other side of the bridge, you will enter

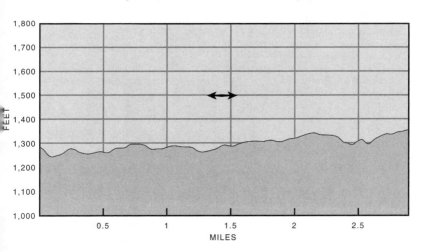

the forest again, where tall pines and hemlocks shade the trail thoroughly. The trail, emblazoned with yellow Department of Environmental Conservation trail markers, is wide and clearly visible among the leaf and needle litter. With few obstructions and roots, typical of most Adirondack trails, the hike is very easygoing. At 0.2 mile, you will pass the trail register, and the forest transitions from mostly conifers to mixed hardwoods. Interspersed with the dominant beech and maple trees are large cherry trees, all of which provide a dense, high canopy. The ground cover is mostly trout lily, and the lack of saplings or brush allows deep views into the surrounding forest. The trail meanders north briefly, and you glimpse Beach Millpond off to your left through a dense stand of hemlocks.

At 1.6 miles, you come to the outflow of an old beaver dam. Planks laid lengthwise help you traverse a few muddy spots and are followed by a log-and-plank bridge. After crossing the bridge, the trail immediately turns east to skirt the edge of the beaver pond. A section of the dam has been breached, so the water is not as high as it might have been. The skeletons of pine trees left standing in what is now less a pond and more a marshland provide a stark contrast to the dense forest that sits atop a slight ridge to your right. You will find some good birding and aquatic wildlife viewing in this area, but I doubt that you will linger long, as mosquitoes and black flies relish in ambushing curious hikers here. The muddiest area of the trail is along this edge, and because the slight ridge restricts the trail, your options for avoiding the muck are limited.

After leaving the beaver dam area, the trail passes through a small meadow and then rises to a more scrubby area where the canopy is significantly more open and lower. This brief foray into an open hilltop setting adds nice variety to the trail's ecological niches. After hopping over a few narrow, seasonal creeks, the trail transitions back to a dense forest where pines are the dominant species. At 2.3 miles, the trail has a small switchback that descends to the confluence of Second Creek and the boulder-strewn Independence River. Another recently constructed log-and-plank bridge crosses Second

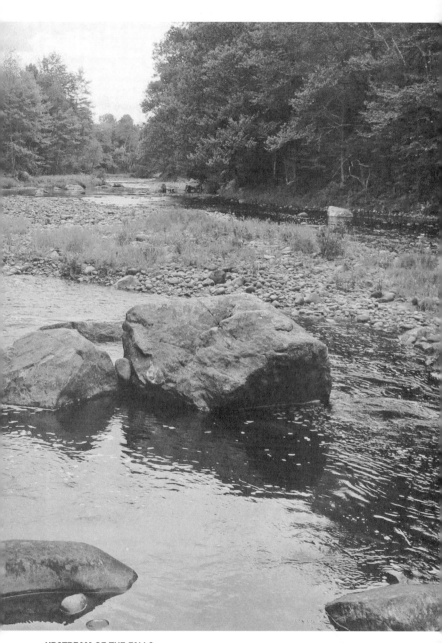

UPSTREAM OF THE FALLS

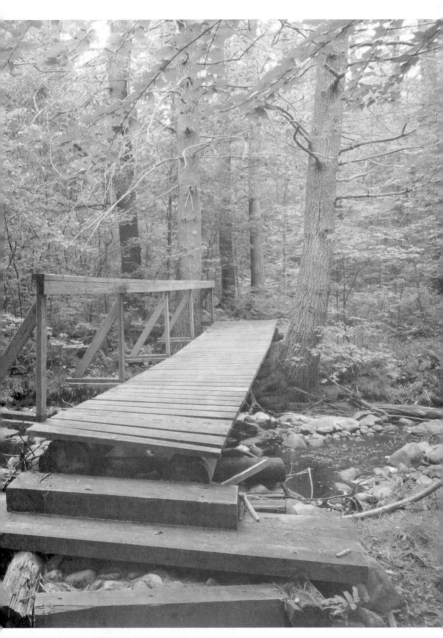

THIS BRIDGE CROSSES OVER A FEEDER STREAM.

Creek, after which the trail climbs slightly over a small hillock dotted with large, moss-covered boulders and then descends to Independence River.

The first of the series of falls is visible here, and a slight scramble to the river's rocky banks will give some glimpses of the falls upriver. You begin to view the roaring falls from atop the narrow gorge after passing a fire pit and informal campsite. These dramatic views of the rushing waters are your true reward and are especially powerful during the spring melts. None of the falls is very tall, but the channeling of the river through this narrow gorge, combined with huge boulders, creates a beautiful scene of cascading and foaming waters. As the trail continues to climb the cliffs alongside the river, the views become more panoramic, with several spectacular views straight down the sheer gorge walls onto the falls. Indeed, the views get successively better along the trail, so do not stop until the trail turns north, back into the forest, around 3 miles. The trail eventually winds back to the river, but the falls will be behind you at this point, and only a scramble back along the rocky wash above the falls will provide any views.

Directions

From NY 12/NY 26/South State Street in Lowville, go east on River Street, which turns into Number Four Road/County Road 22. After 4.3 miles, continue straight onto Pine Grove Road/CR 26. Turn left onto Chase Lake Road after 0.7 mile, 5 miles from Lowville. Continue east along Chase Lake Road, and turn left onto Erie Canal Road in 3.9 miles. Turn right onto Beach Mill Road after 0.6 mile. Continue on the rough and bumpy Beach Mill Road, bearing left at the fork, 1 mile, until the road ends, 3.1 miles.

Central (Hikes 15–23)

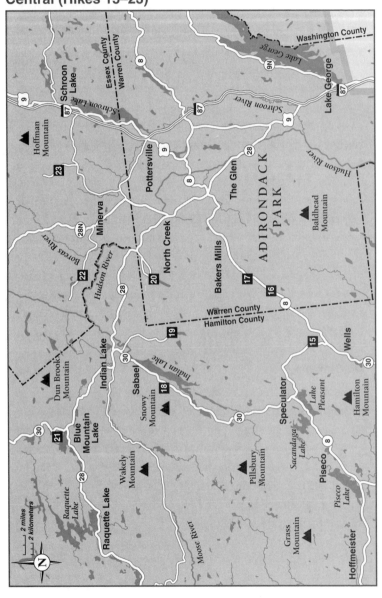

Central

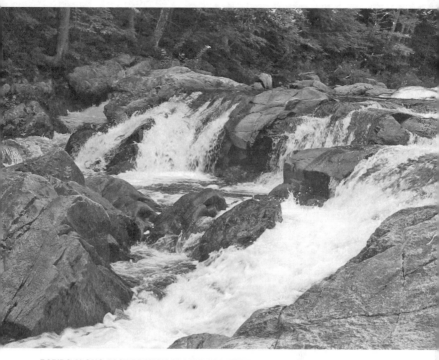

RAPIDS ALONG EAST BRANCH SACANDAGA RIVER *(Trail 17, East Branch Sacandaga Gorge, page 123)*

Auger Falls

SCENERY: ★ ★ ★ ★
TRAIL CONDITION: ★ ★ ★ ★ ★
CHILDREN: ★ ★ ★ ★ ★
DIFFICULTY: ★
SOLITUDE: ★ ★ ★

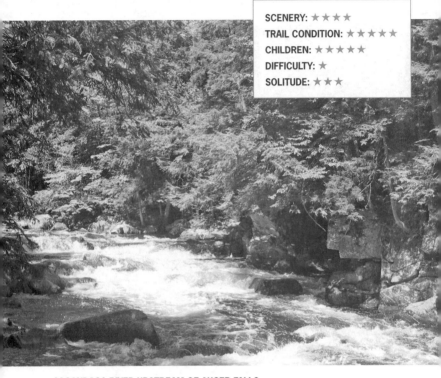

SACANDAGA RIVER UPSTREAM OF AUGER FALLS

GPS COORDINATES: N43° 28.267'   W74° 15.109'

DISTANCE & CONFIGURATION: 1.1-mile loop

HIKING TIME: 1 hour

HIGHLIGHTS: Spectacular waterfall, riverside stroll

ELEVATION: 1,348' at trailhead, with no significant rise

ACCESS: Open 24/7; no fees or permits required

MAPS: National Geographic *Adirondack Park, Northville/Raquette Lake* (#744)

FACILITIES: None

WHEELCHAIR ACCESS: No

CONTACTS: Siamese Ponds Wilderness: www.dec.ny.gov/lands/53172.html; Eastern Adirondack trail information: www.dec.ny.gov/outdoor/9199.html; emergency contact: 518-891-0235

Overview

The powerful falls on the Sacandaga River are truly a sight to see. Channeled into a narrow flume, the river plunges 40 feet in a torrent of foamy waters. As a short-distance loop, this is a great introductory hike for children, but take caution near the falls because the cliffs are steep and potentially slippery.

Route Details

It is easier on your car to park in the large lot that is straight ahead after turning off NY 30. Consequently, directions and mileage are from this point rather than the parking area down the bumpy access road, which is closer to the foot trail's start. From the main parking area, head back toward NY 30, and turn left (southeast) down the access road. Continue down the bumpy, rutted dirt road until you see the Department of Environmental Conservation (DEC) trail sign on your left at 0.3 mile. The trail register is a short distance down the foot trail.

Some people may scoff at the need to sign in for such a short trail, but I encourage hikers to sign in on this and every hike. The DEC and the state base many of their trail-maintenance and funding decisions on trail registers. If you want to see your favorite trails maintained or want more like them, then let the registers act as your democratic voice in the wilderness.

On the trail, walk along the rolling terrain a little more than 0.3 mile through mixed hardwoods. Ahead, you will begin to hear the roar of the falls, and it is likely that you will abandon the trail to explore the numerous paths that diverge from the main trail to find the best vantage point. Many of the paths that offer views and photo ops of the torrential falls are worn and crumbling, so watch your step. The most dramatic part of the waterfall occurs where the river is channeled into a cataract and then plunges down into the gorge formed by the sheer walls of the river. The cliffs on the opposite shore are spectacular, and the dwarfed trees clinging to its ledges only add to the sense of

Auger Falls

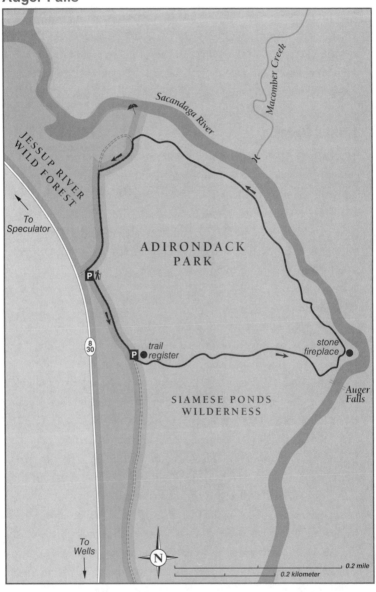

wildness. Photo-worthy views of the opposing sheer cliff and waterfall are found below the falls. Indeed, you can easily reach the middle of the river by hopping along the large boulders that are strewn about at the outwash of the falls. Huge trees lie tangled among the boulders, and it is not hard to picture the powerful flow of water hurling boulders and trees about. To relocate the trail, head back toward the top of the falls, and you will eventually see the yellow disks that mark the trail. It will take you to a beautiful exposed portion of ledge that sits atop the cataract, where an old fireplace has been partially demolished. This spot marks the halfway point and makes an excellent place to stop with the falls thundering below.

To complete the loop, head upstream along the worn, but unmarked, path. Dense conifers crowd the trail in many locations, and you often have to skirt or climb over fallen trees. The calm waters of the river above the falls are a striking contrast to the turbulent waters below. Keep an eye out for a wooden footbridge on the opposite shore, as this indicates that you are nearing the point to turn back west toward the parking area. When you reach a sandy beach near a broad, flat calm in the river, climb over the hillock to your left, and you will come out on the northern end of the parking area.

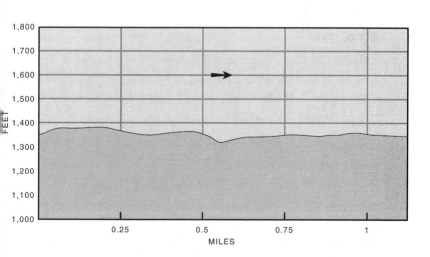

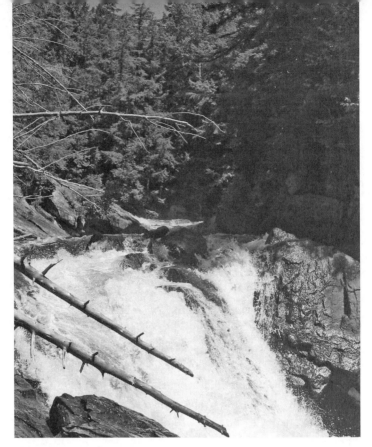

AUGER FALLS

Directions

FROM THE SOUTH   From the intersection of County Road 16 and
NY 30 in Wells, head north on NY 30. At 3.3 miles, bear left to stay
on NY 30/NY 8. At 1.8 miles, turn right onto the unmarked gravel
drive that leads to the parking area.

FROM THE WEST AND NORTH   From the junction of NY 8 and NY
30 in Speculator, continue east on the merged roads NY 30 S/NY 8 N
for 8.2 miles; the unmarked gravel drive will be on the left.

FROM THE EAST   From the junction of NY 8 and NY 30 north of
Wells, turn right onto NY 30/NY 8 toward Speculator. At 1.8 miles, turn
right onto the unmarked gravel drive that leads to the parking area.

Shanty Brook

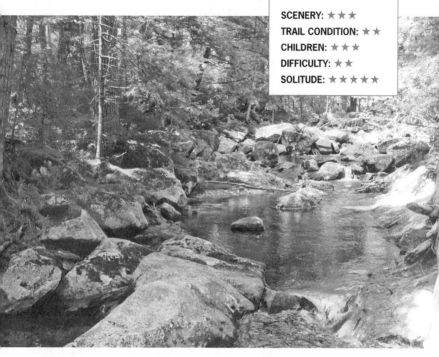

SCENERY: ★ ★ ★
TRAIL CONDITION: ★ ★
CHILDREN: ★ ★ ★
DIFFICULTY: ★ ★
SOLITUDE: ★ ★ ★ ★ ★

SHANTY BROOK SEEN ABOVE THE FALLS

GPS COORDINATES: Parking area: N43° 32.131' W74° 08.487'
Trailhead: N43° 32.258' W74° 8.447'

DISTANCE & CONFIGURATION: 7.6-mile out-and-back

HIKING TIME: 4–5 hours

HIGHLIGHTS: Waterfall, swimming hole, remote pond

ELEVATION: 1,387' at trailhead, 1,693' at highest point

ACCESS: Open 24/7; no fees or permits required

MAPS: National Geographic *Adirondack Park, Northville/Raquette Lake* (#744)

FACILITIES: None

WHEELCHAIR ACCESS: No

CONTACTS: Siamese Ponds Wilderness: www.dec.ny.gov/lands/53172.html; Eastern
Adirondack trail information: www.dec.ny.gov/outdoor/9199.html; emergency contact:
518-891-0235

Shanty Brook

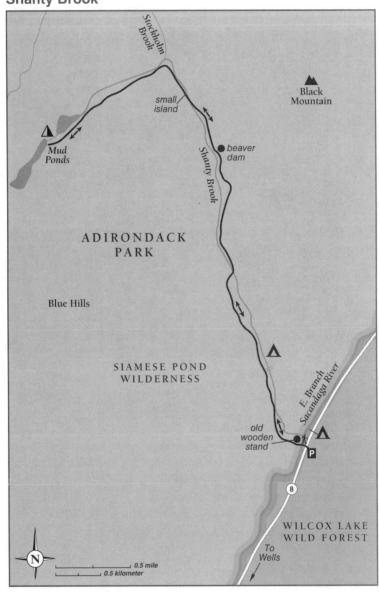

Overview

Though not difficult, this unmarked trail varies from a narrow footpath to an outright bushwhack, so unseasoned hikers should be prepared before undertaking this adventure. One of the more notable preparations is to expect to have wet feet. There is almost no getting around this, so plan accordingly, and you will be able to enjoy the beautiful waterfall, swimming hole, and remote pond.

Route Details

Most of the parking areas along NY 8 are unmarked, so finding the right one can be tricky. Fortunately, paying attention to your odometer readings and your GPS should steer you in the right direction. The parking area for Shanty Brook is distinct because it is on the south side of the road and is the only one that is U-shaped; most are large lots or gravel pulloffs right next to the road. The trail is unmarked, and though portions are well worn, this hike definitely counts as a bushwhack. You have to wade across the East Branch of the Sacandaga River, so either bring water shoes or plan to hike in wet boots. Additionally, the rocks in the river are slippery, so you will appreciate having a change of clothes in a dry sack should the crossing not go according to plan.

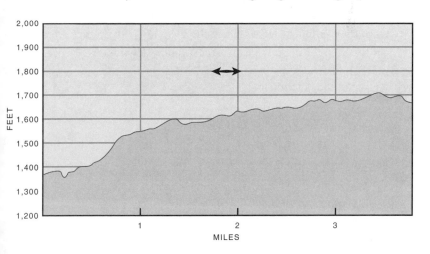

To reach the river crossing, head northeast along NY 8 a few hundred feet to where a short dirt road provides access to a designated campsite along the river. A steep drop-off leads down to the East Branch of the Sacandaga River on the left side of the road. Across the river, you will see where Shanty Brook meets the river, and you should start looking for a good crossing point. The trail is on the west side of the brook, and I found that an easy way down to the river is about midway down the road, where an old wooden stand once provided access to a cable crossing. The cable crossing was removed, but the stand remains a good landmark. This is less than 100 feet downriver from the confluence of the brook and river. On the opposite shore, you can see where the vegetation has been beaten down where the cable used to be connected. Carefully wade across the river, or rock-hop if the season has been dry enough; do not count on keeping your feet dry.

On the opposite shore, a well-worn path leads to the western bank of the brook. The trail parallels the brook and crosses several muddy sections as you begin a gentle climb. A little less than 0.8 mile in, you will see a path to your right and notice that the rumble of the brook has gotten louder. Follow the path to the right to reach the top of the waterfall. The falls plunge 12 feet, though they seem taller, into a deep pool that is enclosed within the steep banks of the brook. To reach the base of the waterfall and the swimming hole, jump across the brook to the opposite shore, and scramble down the banks over roots and rocks to the base of the falls. The pool at the base of the falls is not large but is deep enough to swim in, and you can swim right into the falls. A little upstream on the east shore is a designated campsite that would be ideal for a short overnight trip.

Back along the main trail, the path climbs a bit more but quickly levels off for most of the rest of the trip. A quarter mile from the falls, the trail veers away from the brook but then turns briefly east and crosses the brook 0.8 mile from the falls, 1.5 miles from the start. You will pass an open area and beaver dam along the brook at approximately 2.3 miles. This is the first of two open areas along

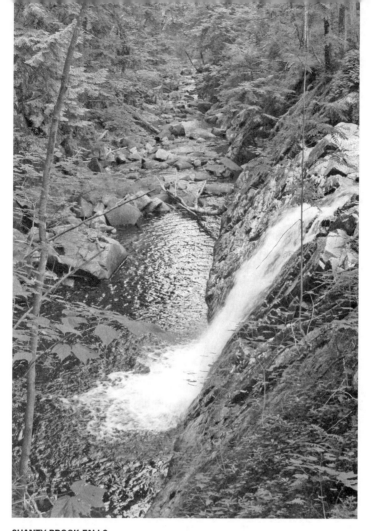

SHANTY BROOK FALLS

the brook that provide views of the surrounding hills. At the second open area, 2.6 miles, the trail seems to abruptly terminate in a sandy wash. The meadow lies straight before you, rather than to your left as it was previously. This is where you need to recross the brook to reach Mud Ponds. The path on the opposite shore is hard to discern in the summer growth and flooded-out areas, but as long as you keep the brook on your right, you will eventually find a well-worn section of the path. I found that by following a small seasonal channel between an evergreen-dotted island on your right and the surrounding hill-side to your left, you can more easily work your way north to the more distinct portions of the path.

The trail from this point on is not traveled as heavily, and blow-down and washouts make navigating a little more difficult. Hikers who are not familiar with basic navigation, lack a compass and map or a good sense of direction, or are uncomfortable with unmarked trails would probably be better served returning before the crossing instead of finishing the hike to Mud Ponds. If you choose to continue, gaiters provide a welcome reprieve from the leg lashings of brambles and fallen trees that encroach on the trail.

A third of a mile from the recrossing, 3 miles from the start, the trail swings west as you follow Shanty Brook, now on your right, toward Mud Ponds. The brook now flows over mostly level ground and is much more placid than before. At 3.2 miles, you reach what appears to be the eastern tip of Mud Ponds, but it is only a widening of the brook due to beaver activity. The actual eastern tip is at 3.6 miles. The path weaves its way along the southern shore of the pond through thick overgrowth and wet sections. At 3.7 miles, you pass a grassy channel that connects the two main ponds and soon reach a small hill that lies between the ponds. Atop this hill is an informal campsite with benches and a fire pit, which, for all intents and purposes, marks the end of the bushwhack. Farther on are more paths, but they soon end in impassable brambles or mires.

Directions

From the intersection of NY 30 and NY 8 in Wells, follow NY 8 north-east 8.9 miles. The parking area is on your right in the shape of a U.

From the intersection of NY 28 and NY 8 in Wevertown, follow NY 8 west 14.5 miles. The parking area is on your left in the shape of a U.

East Branch Sacandaga Gorge

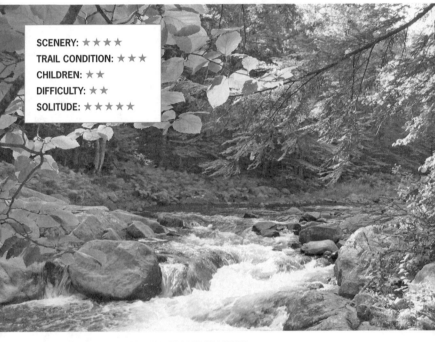

SCENERY: ★ ★ ★ ★
TRAIL CONDITION: ★ ★ ★
CHILDREN: ★ ★
DIFFICULTY: ★ ★
SOLITUDE: ★ ★ ★ ★ ★

RAPIDS ON THE EAST BRANCH SACANDAGA RIVER

GPS COORDINATES: N43° 34.146'   W74° 06.798'

DISTANCE & CONFIGURATION: 2.4-mile loop or out-and-back

HIKING TIME: 1–2 hours

HIGHLIGHTS: Waterfall, swimming hole, scenic river gorge

ELEVATION: 1,435' at trailhead, 1,510' at highest point

ACCESS: Open 24/7; no fees or permits required

MAPS: National Geographic *Adirondack Park, Northville/Raquette Lake* (#744)

FACILITIES: None

WHEELCHAIR ACCESS: No

CONTACTS: Siamese Ponds Wilderness: www.dec.ny.gov/lands/53172.html; Eastern Adirondack trail information: www.dec.ny.gov/outdoor/9199.html; emergency contact: 518-891-0235

East Branch Sacandaga Gorge

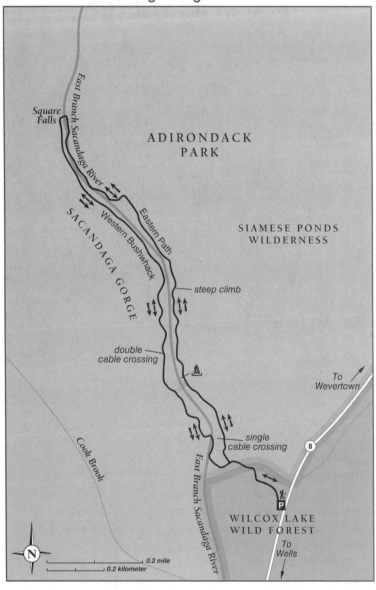

Overview

The East Branch of the Sacandaga River has a spectacular gorge with a serene waterfall and swimming hole that you can reach in two ways. The most direct and clearest route is to follow the eastern footpath to Square Falls. The most scenic and adventurous route is to ford the river and then bushwhack along the western banks. Neither route is very long, and the two are easily combined if you choose to ford the river twice.

Route Details

There are no trail signs or indications of the trailhead either in the expansive parking area or from NY 8, so pay attention to your odometer, as there are numerous unmarked parking areas along NY 8. Additionally, there is no trail register, and the trail is not marked, but if you pay attention to the directions below, the paths are fairly easy to find and follow. The trail begins on the northeastern edge of the parking area along an old road. The abandoned dirt road descends generally northwest from the main road into the forest. Approximately 0.1 mile down, you reach the end of the road and a turnaround on your left. Large boulders on your right barricade the remaining trail from

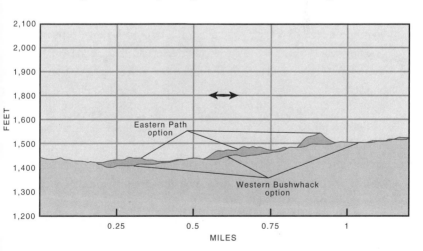

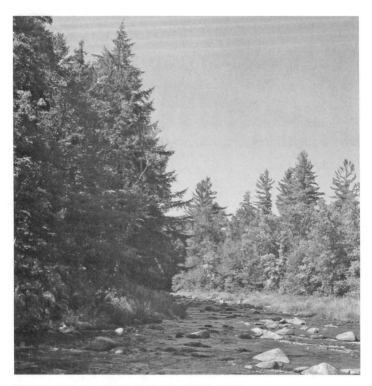

EAST BRANCH SACANDAGA RIVER BELOW THE GORGE

vehicular travel. Wind your way down the trail to the small stream crossing shortly ahead. Once across the stream, you must decide which route you will choose to explore the gorge. The path along the eastern edge is hard to make out amid the debris of seasonal flooding but is easily distinguished by climbing the tiny hill directly to your right. The western bushwhack is accessed by continuing straight ahead and then heading toward the river along numerous footpaths. Both options, described separately below, terminate at Square Falls, where you can easily ford the river if you wish to combine the trips. If you choose to take the eastern path and return along the western edge, then you should scope out the condition of the river now before continuing. There are two reasons to do so: First, you will need to recognize where to recross the river; second, you will need to determine whether the river is shallow enough to rock-hop or if wading in the strong current will be necessary. Upriver, several narrow areas make crossing easier.

Eastern Path

Following the eastern path is by far the easiest, safest, and fastest approach to the falls. If it were not for the dramatic scenery offered along the western bushwhack and the lack of scenery on this bank, I would recommend this route to all hikers. Once you're on this well-trodden path, it is hard to lose. For the most part, the path winds atop the gorge cliffs, so views of the river and the dramatic walls are obscured by dense foliage below, but the torrent of water can be heard most of the way. Roughly 0.3 mile in, you arrive at the cascade at the end of the gorge, where an old fire pit is situated close to the riverbank. A tenth of a mile ahead, you pass the double-cable crossing described below. At 0.6 mile, the trail climbs very steeply away from the banks, and you walk high above the river 0.3 mile before winding your way back down to the river. You have passed the gorge portion of the hike, but the falls and swimming hole await you 0.3 mile ahead. The river is visible along this last portion of the trail and makes for some beautiful scenery, but this route has nowhere near the dramatic contrasts of the western bushwhack.

Western Bushwhack

If you choose this option instead of the eastern path, upon reaching the banks of the East Branch of the Sacandaga River, you will face the decision of where to cross. Only hikers who are nimble and willing to wade should attempt the crossing. Rock-hopping is a better choice and might get you across (or, as I found, most of the way across) with short sections remaining to be waded. Despite appearing relatively flat, the current is strong, and the round rocks that line the riverbed are slick with slime, so be mindful of your footing. Now that the caveats have been established, let us recognize that in summer, wading across the river can be quite fun and refreshing. Besides, you are headed to a swimming hole. I found an easily recognizable section to cross upriver where two large boulders sit on the southern bank.

Once on the opposite bank, the path is not readily clear, but rest assured that you will find it if you head upriver close to the rocky banks. Hemlock saplings crowd the banks, while mature trees shade the west side of the river. The informal path on this side of the river is distinct in some areas and disappears among the dense saplings and fallen trees in others, but if you keep the river within sight on your right, you will find your way to the falls. Roughly 0.3 mile into the hike, the gorge begins with a small cascade among the boulder-strewn banks. As you hike, you will notice that the bank on the eastern side is nearly vertical; in sections it ranges from 50 to 100 feet high, and with the frothy water churning beneath, the scenery has a distinctly wild and rugged character. Approximately 0.5 mile into the hike, the steep riverbanks draw close together, with a nearly 20-foot drop to the river. A double cable strung between large eastern white pines on the opposing banks provides a crossing over a deep pool. I don't recommend this crossing except for experienced hikers who have a means to tie off and are in the company of other hikers. Above the pool, the river contracts to a narrow flume through which it spurts out a torrent of foam. You will pass several other small cascades on your way upriver, all of which may seem like Square Falls. However, you won't reach Square Falls until you have hiked 1.2 miles; you can distinguish it from the other cascades because it forms a 6- to 8-foot cascade across the entire river. Additionally, a wide pool lies at its base, while a broad, tabular portion of bedrock forms its top.

Directions

From the intersection of NY 30 and NY 8 in Wells, travel east on NY 8. The parking area is 11.7 miles ahead on your left.

From the intersection of NY 28 and NY 8 in Wevertown, head west on NY 8. The parking area is 11.7 miles ahead on your right.

Snowy Mountain

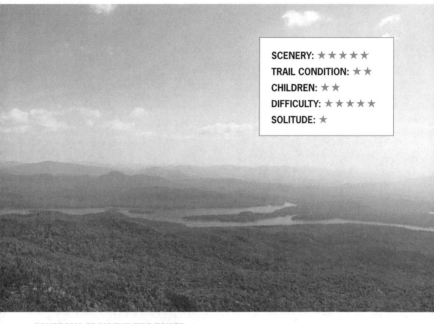

SCENERY: ★ ★ ★ ★ ★
TRAIL CONDITION: ★ ★
CHILDREN: ★ ★
DIFFICULTY: ★ ★ ★ ★ ★
SOLITUDE: ★

PANORAMA FROM THE FIRE TOWER

GPS COORDINATES: N43° 42.081' W74° 20.090'

DISTANCE & CONFIGURATION: 7.4-mile out-and-back

HIKING TIME: 4.5–5.5 hours

HIGHLIGHTS: Panoramic views, accessible fire tower

ELEVATION: 1,807' at trailhead, 3,899' at Snowy Mountain peak

ACCESS: Open 24/7; no fees or permits required

MAPS: National Geographic *Adirondack Park, Northville/Raquette Lake* (#744)

FACILITIES: None

WHEELCHAIR ACCESS: No

COMMENTS: The trail signs indicate that the distance to the peak is 3.4 miles, but the actual distance is closer to 3.7 miles. The final ascent is very steep and difficult, so plan accordingly and take your time.

CONTACTS: Central and Southern Adirondack trail information: www.dec.ny.gov/outdoor /9200.html; emergency contact: 518-891-0235

Snowy Mountain

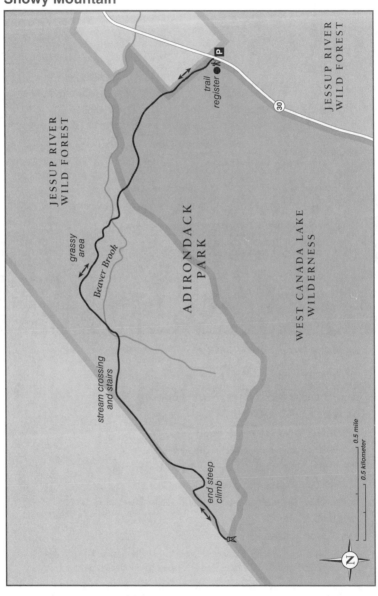

Overview

Snowy Mountain is considered by many as the 47th High Peak, even though at 3,899 feet tall, it falls just under the 4,000-foot threshold to be considered one of the famous 46 High Peaks. However, recent surveys have shown that 4 of the 46 peaks are under 4,000 feet and 2 (Nye Mountain and Couchsachraga) are actually shorter than Snowy Mountain. Unlike many mountain hikes featured in the book, this is not one of the "bald" peaks that provide the awe-inspiring views for which the Adirondack mountaintops are famous. But just because it is not a bald peak does not mean the mountain is short on views. Indeed there are a couple of stunning lookouts near the peak, but the real gem is the 360-degree panorama atop the 45-foot-tall accessible fire tower.

Route Details

Parking along the eastern side of NY 30 is more than adequate for a dozen cars or more, but the trail is so popular that often dozens more line the road to the north and south of the parking area. The assemblage of vehicles is actually a useful landmark as the trail sign/trailhead is often obscured by the thick foliage along the west side of

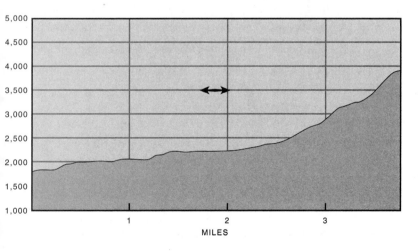

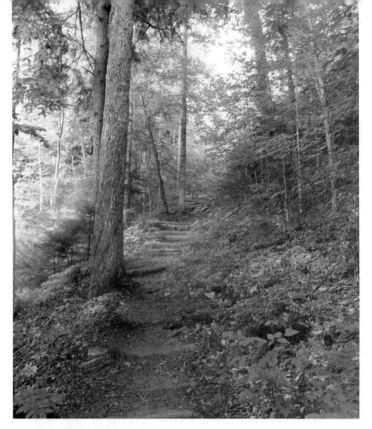

LOG STAIRS MAKE THE CLIMB EASIER.

the road. The trailhead is nearly directly opposite the pulloff/parking area, and you find the trail register just beyond the thick vegetation.

The trail, marked with red trail markers, heads briefly uphill and then begins a 1-mile, relatively flat course (200' elevation gain) west through deciduous forest. Along the way it crosses several small, seasonal brooks and traverses several wet areas atop zigzagged planks. Beaver Brook soon becomes visible down to the right, but there is one more seasonal brook crossing before you descend to the first of several crossings of Beaver Brook, indicated here by a painted arrow sign.

Rock-hop across, and climb the opposite bank. After briefly navigating a wet area over a corduroy bridge, the trail diverges from Beaver Brook and begins a modest climb (roughly 200 feet over the next 0.25 mile). Log steps cut into the earth assist you along this climb, after which the trail levels off. At 1.5 miles from the trailhead, a placid creek bisects the trail in an open, marshy area. Cross along the log-and-plank bridge, and continue 0.4 mile along level ground to where you intersect Beaver Brook again.

The trail begins a steady climb west as you crisscross Beaver Brook over the next 0.5 mile, and you will have to pick your way carefully through several long, boot-sucking mires as you ascend beside the brook. The final crossing of Beaver Brook, roughly 2.5 miles from the trailhead, is distinct from other crossings in that stone steps beckon you forward on the southern bank. The steps also allude to the increasing grade of the climb ahead (nearly 1,500 feet in less than 1.25 miles).

At this point the trail has covered roughly two-thirds of the distance to the peak but only one-third of the elevation gain. The grade grows steadily steeper and requires using your hands to climb as you near the peak. About 0.75 mile ahead, the trail swings nearly due south and there is a brief slackening of the grade and short respite along the climb. This relatively flat section of trail lies within an evergreen stand and is a good stopping point to get ready for the even steeper portions ahead. Whereas the trail had gained roughly 800 feet over the previous 0.75 mile, along the next section, the trail gains 600 feet in less than 0.3 mile.

The new ascent begins as the trail swings more westerly, but calling parts of the next section "a trail" is a bit misleading because the path soon becomes what is actually a jumble and wash of large boulders and an inclined ledge so broad that the canopy gives way to the open sky. Some portions have no defined route and will likely require the use of both hands as you climb. Follow this open swath upward, picking your way carefully through the vertical maze of rocks. At the top is a small, flat area where you can pause before continuing on to the last bit of climbing. Bear right (west) and begin the final ascent (200 feet) that ends after you pass a sheer rock wall on the right and reaches the first of two lookouts found near the peak.

The first lookout is to the right of the trail in an open field with a steep ledge you can sit on along the northern edge. Other hikers are likely to congregate here because it is a better place to stop and rest before beginning your descent than the actual peak and fire tower less than 0.1 mile ahead.

The second lookout is along the western edge of the peak and is more isolated and private. To reach it, you will have to follow some of the unmarked footpaths that weave and meander across the peak; to find the right one, bear right off the main trail onto one of these paths, and you should find it easily. The lookout is atop an exposed ledge, encircled by stubby evergreens, that has an almost perfect natural bench on which to sit in relative solitude and take in the view. However, depending on the time of year, this area may be a bit buggy on calm days.

As it is for most hikers, the fire tower is likely your ultimate destination and can be found by following the footpaths that lead south over a couple of short hillocks. The actual highest point of the peak lies here, but the peak is heavily wooded, so vistas are available only to those who climb the extra 45 feet to the top of the tower. Like the other fire towers that dot the Adirondack peaks, space within the tower is limited, so hikers will have to take turns inside. Because the stairs are narrow, without much room to pass, it is best to let previous occupants come back down before trying to climb up.

Directions

FROM THE SOUTH   From the intersection of NY 8 and NY 30 in Speculator, head north along NY 30. Continue 17.1 miles; the pulloff will be on the right.

FROM THE NORTh   From the intersection of NY 28 and NY 30 in Indian Lake, head south along NY 30. Continue 7.3 miles; the pulloff will be on the left.

Chimney Mountain

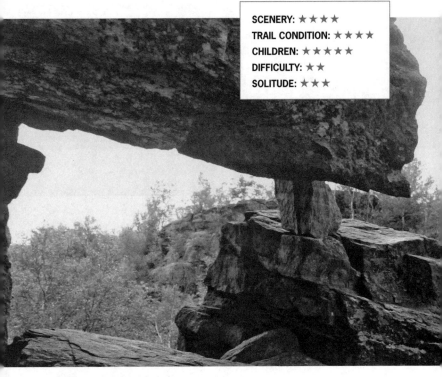

SCENERY: ★ ★ ★ ★
TRAIL CONDITION: ★ ★ ★ ★
CHILDREN: ★ ★ ★ ★ ★
DIFFICULTY: ★ ★
SOLITUDE: ★ ★ ★

THE WINDOW AT CHIMNEY MOUNTAIN

GPS COORDINATES: N43° 41.289'   W74° 13.809'

DISTANCE & CONFIGURATION: 2.2-mile out-and-back

HIKING TIME: 1 hour

HIGHLIGHTS: Interesting geological formations

ELEVATION: 1,751' at trailhead, 2,703' at highest point

ACCESS: Open 24/7; no permits required; $2 parking fee

MAPS: National Geographic *Adirondack Park, Northville/Raquette Lake* (#744)

FACILITIES: None

WHEELCHAIR ACCESS: No

CONTACTS: Siamese Ponds Wilderness: www.dec.ny.gov/lands/53172.html; Eastern Adirondack trail information: www.dec.ny.gov/outdoor/9199.html; emergency contact: 518-891-0131

Chimney Mountain

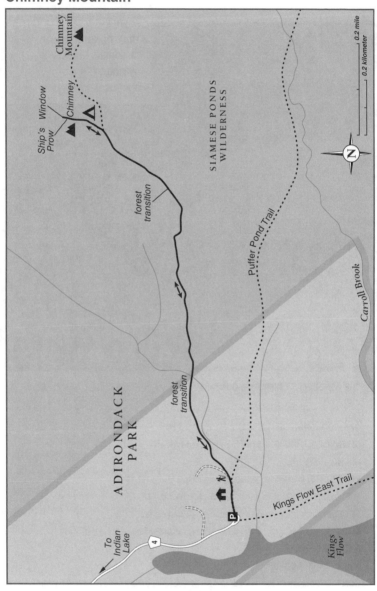

Overview

In a region noted for beautiful lakes and panoramic mountains, this geological oddity adds a spectacular variation. Formed over millennia, Chimney Mountain provides a great opportunity to view the geological forces that shaped the Adirondacks. Exploring the numerous formations will occupy most for hours, but for the spelunker and amateur geologist, a day trip probably will not suffice.

Route Details

The parking area for Chimney Mountain, as well as Puffer Pond and Kings Flow East Trails, is on private land, with a day-use fee of $2 per car. Many of Adirondack Park's best hikes and features are available through cooperation between private landholders and the Department of Environmental Conservation (DEC). To ensure this cooperation and to encourage future collaborations, please respect private property, and pay the day-use fee.

To reach the trailhead, walk up the gravel drive past several cabins, approximately 0.2 mile from the parking area. The register is located beneath the shade of the encompassing forest. The Puffer Pond and Kings Flow East Trailheads are to your right, while the

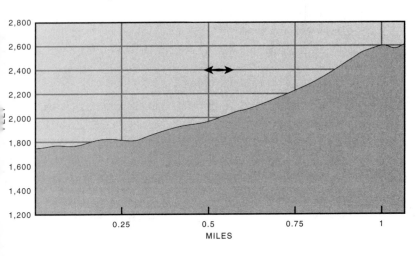

Chimney Mountain Trail is to your left. Trail maps often show the two sharing a section of the trail, but the portion shared is actually the access road before the trail register. Mileage given is from the actual trailhead and not from the parking area.

Passing through a thick band of saplings along the forest's edge, you will quickly notice that the trail is wide, well worn, and easy to follow. Blue DEC disks mark the trail but are hardly necessary except near the top, where numerous paths lead to caves and other geological points of interest. Shrouded in tall hardwoods, most notably birches and maples, the trail is fairly level until 0.2 mile, where you cross a brook and the climbing begins. The grade is moderate at first but steadily increases toward the peak. The forest eventually transitions from the deep woodlands to a more open and parklike setting approximately 0.7 mile along. On steeper sections of the trail, take a look back, and you will see Round Lake, which seems to hover at the bases of Crotched Pond Mountain and Kunjamuk Mountain.

Closer to the summit, you will begin encountering informal paths that wind off to your left. This maze of paths leads to some lesser rock formations, to numerous crevices and caves, and to another elevated ridge from which you can look back at the chimney. The caves have precipitous drops, so be cautious when off the main trail, especially with curious and bold children. Exploring the caves should be left to people who are properly experienced and equipped. Do not attempt these activities if you are a novice. However, there are plenty of wonders and much to explore along the main trail, so don't feel like you are missing out if you do not explore off the trail.

The spire, an amalgamation of metamorphosed rocks, will begin to tower ahead and draw you through ledges that flank the trail. The marked trail ends here, but do not let that stop you from scrambling among the rocks. Just be cautious near the northern edge, as the drop-off is precipitous. The convoluted layers of different materials will likely raise an eyebrow as you puzzle over how such rocks come into being. See page 1 for an elementary description. The story of these epoch transformations is revealed in the exposed portions of Chimney Mountain.

A description of all the interesting formations and ways to find and explore them is beyond the scope of this book and, frankly, this author. However, I will name a couple that you can easily and safely access from the main trail. The main passage you encounter has the jumble of rocks that make up the Chimney to your left and a narrow ledge called the Ship's Prow. The prow is easily walkable, but it narrows and the fall is more precipitous as you go—know your limits before attempting to walk to its end. Turning left at the trail's end, you walk under a striking overhang and come out with the Chimney looming to your right. Climbing along its base to the opposite side will reveal the Window; it frames the western ledge and is easy to crawl into. In addition to the formations, various points offer panoramic views of the ridge to the west, as well as seemingly endless peaks in every direction.

Chances are that as you looked up onto the spire when you climbed, you missed a path to the right, which leads to an informal campsite. As you leave the Chimney, this path is more obvious off to your left. Just past the campsite, the path leads not only to the actual summit of Chimney Mountain but also to an interesting view through the surrounding trees of Ship's Prow with the Chimney towering behind it.

Directions

From the intersection of NY 30 and NY 28 in Indian Lake, head south on NY 30. Turn left onto County Road 4/Big Brook Road at 0.6 mile. Follow Big Brook Road across Lake Abanakee, and take a sharp right at 6.1 miles. At 7.8 miles park in the designated parking area and pay the day-use fee.

Peaked Mountain

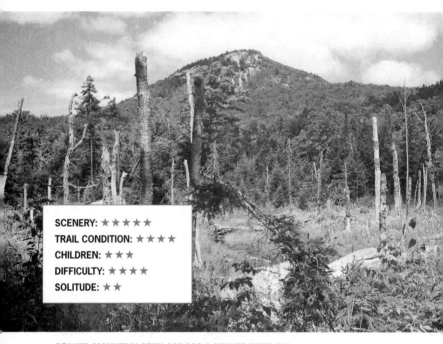

SCENERY: ★ ★ ★ ★ ★
TRAIL CONDITION: ★ ★ ★ ★
CHILDREN: ★ ★ ★
DIFFICULTY: ★ ★ ★ ★
SOLITUDE: ★ ★

PEAKED MOUNTAIN SEEN ACROSS A BEAVER MEADOW

GPS COORDINATES: N43° 43.125'   W74° 07.110'

DISTANCE & CONFIGURATION: 7.2-mile out-and-back

HIKING TIME: 4 hours

HIGHLIGHTS: Lakeside hiking, cascades along a stream, beaver dams and meadows, isolated pond, panoramic views from a peak

ELEVATION: 1,726' at trailhead, 2,919' at highest point

ACCESS: Open 24/7; no fees or permits required

MAPS: National Geographic *Adirondack Park, Northville/Raquette Lake* (#744)

FACILITIES: None

WHEELCHAIR ACCESS: Accessible campsites and bathrooms are at Thirteenth Lake.

CONTACTS: Siamese Ponds Wilderness: www.dec.ny.gov/lands/53172.html; Eastern Adirondack trail information: www.dec.ny.gov/outdoor/9199.html; emergency contact: 518-891-0235

Overview

Can't choose between lakeside hiking, exploring an isolated pond, hiking beside frothy cascades, or climbing a mountain for a panoramic view? Why choose? Peaked Mountain has it all. The main trail is easy and features a variety of waterscapes, including a pristine lake, a cascading brook, and several beaver dam meadows. The last 0.8 mile along the trail is steep and difficult, but the summit has a unique perspective. At the peak, you can clearly trace your entire trip back to the shore of Thirteenth Lake.

Route Details

Access to Peaked Mountain is at the north end of Thirteenth Lake, which also has car-top boat access, accessible picnic areas, and free primitive camping. Most of the vehicles in the large and spacious parking area are for camping and day use. To access the trail, walk down the main gravel drive to the trail register. The register also serves as a record of day-use activities, so do not be surprised to see a lot of entries. To the left is the boat launch, while access to the foot trail is down the right fork. Head toward the lake past a couple of campsites and picnic tables, and then look for the trail sign on your right near the last picnic table. Mileage given is from this point, which is a little more than 0.1 mile from the parking area.

The trail winds along the shore of Thirteenth Lake, weaving through paper birches and other hardwoods. Beaver activity is evident everywhere, from chewed stumps and recently felled trees across the path to several lodges that are within feet of the trail. The trail is relatively flat, with a few dips and hills that follow the contours of the lake. You will encounter a couple of designated primitive campsites along the trail as well, so be aware that you may be walking through or near someone's site.

The shores of Thirteenth Lake are undeveloped and pristine. Though not common, motorboaters are occasionally heard, which is odd because the lake is nestled in the middle of a wilderness area.

Peaked Mountain

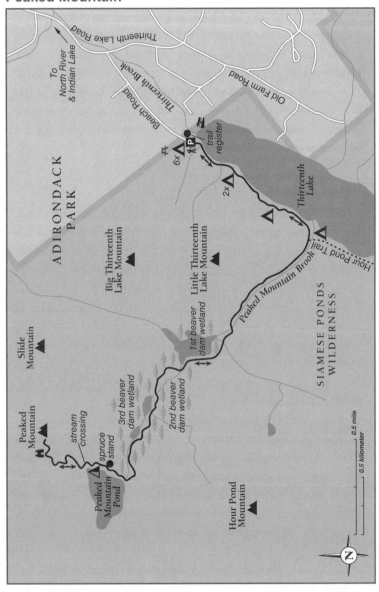

(Wilderness Area land-use plans typically prohibit the use of motorized boats; hopefully the state will enforce this standard in the future.) Typically, the lake is dotted with canoeists and kayakers, and in fact, many of these boaters paddle to where the trail diverges from the lake, around 0.8 mile on the right.

This junction occurs where Peaked Mountain Brook empties into Thirteenth Lake. Shortly after you begin following the brook uphill, you encounter a trail sign indicating Hour Pond to your left. However, to reach Peaked Mountain and its pond, continue northwest uphill alongside the brook. You will be following Peaked Mountain Brook through numerous transformations all the way to the pond and the foot of the mountain. Innumerable small falls and cascades characterize the brook until you cross it upstream, at 1.5 miles, and provide an interesting contrast to the flat and quiet waters of the lake behind you. You will have to rock-hop across the brook to a tiny island and then again to the opposite bank.

The trail levels off after crossing the brook. Shortly after, you will notice a clearing to your right, a result of the first dammed section of the brook. From the trail, hemlocks frame the grassy wetland and an outstanding view of Slide Mountain. Farther along, the trail winds closer to the wetland, and looking east, you will see Big Thirteenth

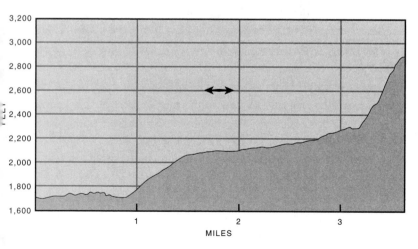

MILES

Lake Mountain. This is the first of three distinct beaver-dammed sections along the brook, but with all the evident beaver activity, the landscape could easily change from year to year. It is tempting to think that one of these dammed sections is Peaked Mountain Pond and that one of the mountains is Peaked Mountain. However, the pond is a broader expanse of still water, and Peaked Mountain has exposed sheer faces with less tree cover.

After looking across the wetland at Big Thirteenth Lake Mountain, you will pass very close to a large beaver dam at 1.9 miles. Shortly after, you cross the brook again and head back into the woods briefly before another wetland opens up to your left. A couple of rocks along the trail's edge provide a good vantage point of the dammed wetland, which surrounds a tiny, cedar-dotted island. The trail hugs the eastern edge of this wetland and then recrosses Peaked Mountain Brook at the northern edge of the wetland. The crossing is little more than a step across the brook, where it passes between two broad rocks, and you are roughly two-thirds of the way to the pond. The third and final major dammed section gives you the first real glimpse of Peaked Mountain's large, exposed face. This section contains a lot more large dead trees, with the additional distinction of large boulders strewn about.

After a short section of walking through dense woods, you climb a small hill to discover Peaked Mountain Pond straight ahead at 3 miles. At this point, paths lead off to your left, but the trail is to your right. A fallen tree makes this a convenient spot to sit next to the pond. However, a nice place to rest is also a little farther up the trail in a small area of spruces. The trail so far has been fairly easy and accessible to most hikers. However, the climb to the summit is much steeper and requires a lot more effort. It is certainly worth the ascent, so take time to rest and enjoy the view of the beautiful pond.

The trail up the mountain passes through the previously mentioned stand of spruces and past a fork in the trail, which indicates a designated camping area to the left. The trail climbs slightly, among beeches and maples, and then descends to a stream crossing with views of the pond to your left. Climbing begins immediately after

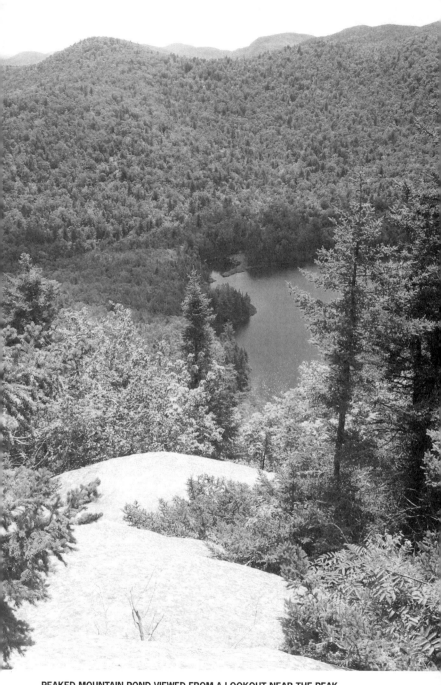

PEAKED MOUNTAIN POND VIEWED FROM A LOOKOUT NEAR THE PEAK

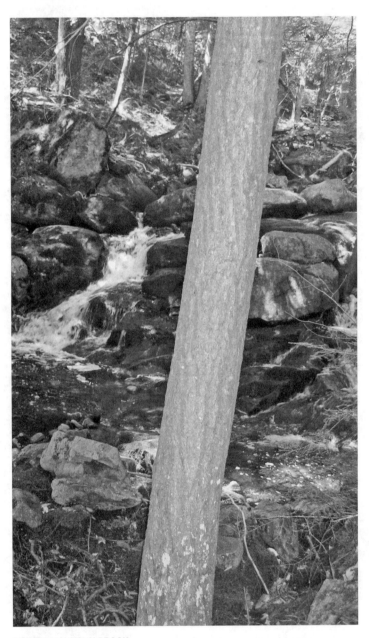

PEAKED MOUNTAIN BROOK

you cross the stream. This section is steep, with large, exposed rocks, and the forest is almost entirely paper birches. Blown-down birches often cover the trail, making spotting the actual trail and finding the best footing difficult at times. However, red disks mark the trail, and alternate paths around the blowdown are evident.

After the first steep section, the grade eases a bit through a section where sheer rock is on your left and a rock hump is to your right. The trail swings left just past a massive boulder and becomes steep again. Climbing is steady until just before the top, and there are several tricky spots, so take your time and make room for other hikers as they pass. When evergreens dominate the forest, you'll know that you are close to the summit. A large, open portion of bedrock provides views down onto the pond, but the best part is at the true summit. After a brief foray back into the evergreens, you are once again out in the open. Sprawling out beneath you is your entire trip from where you left Thirteenth Lake. Peaked Mountain Pond and the beaver-dammed sections are obvious, as is the path the brook has cut into the landscape. In the height of summer, dragonflies perform aerial acrobatics for your viewing pleasure, and the bedrock provides a great spot to sit and look out at the beautiful vista.

Directions

FROM THE WEST   From the intersection of NY 28 and NY 30 in Indian Lake, head 12.1 miles east along NY 28, and turn right onto County Road 78/Thirteenth Lake Road in North River. Bear right onto Beach Road at 3.3 miles. End at the large parking area at 0.7 mile.

FROM THE EAST   From the intersection of NY 28 and NY 28N in North Creek, head 5.2 miles west along NY 28. Turn left onto CR 78/Thirteenth Lake Road. Bear right onto Beach Road at 3.3 miles. End at the large parking area at 0.7 mile.

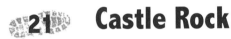

Castle Rock

SCENERY: ★ ★ ★	
TRAIL CONDITION: ★ ★ ★	
CHILDREN: ★ ★ ★ ★ ★	
DIFFICULTY: ★ ★	
SOLITUDE: ★ ★ ★ ★ ★	

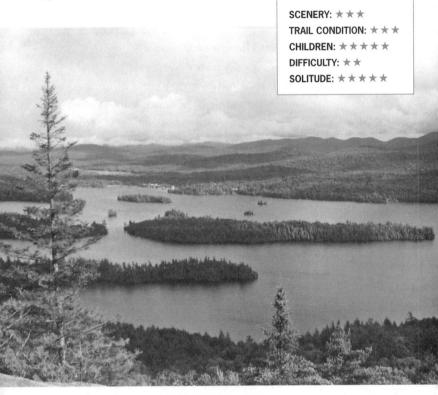

BLUE MOUNTAIN LAKE SEEN FROM CASTLE ROCK

GPS COORDINATES: N43° 52.370'   W74° 27.071'

DISTANCE & CONFIGURATION: 3.7-mile loop

HIKING TIME: 2 hours

HIGHLIGHTS: Scenic views, cliffs

ELEVATION: 1,880' at trailhead, 2,430' at highest point

ACCESS: Open 24/7; no fees or permits required

MAPS: National Geographic *Adirondack Park, Northville/Raquette Lake* (#744)

FACILITIES: None

WHEELCHAIR ACCESS: No

CONTACTS: Central and Southern Adirondack trail information: www.dec.ny.gov/outdoor /9200.html; emergency contact: 518-891-0235

Overview

From a glance at a map, this trail looks deceptively uninteresting, but it has a lot to keep your attention. The analogy to a castle is well founded, and those with active imaginations will find themselves naming gates, turrets, and other structures while exploring the area. As a short loop, it provides a refreshing change from the innumerable out-and-backs typical of summits and other trails in the park.

Route Details

The parking area is a small pulloff near the Minnowbrook Conference Center. The trail register is just up the road within sight of the sandy parking area. However, the trail does not begin until a little more than 0.3 mile down the road. Mileage given here is from the trail register. Follow the private gravel road, and bear right where the conference center driveway rejoins the road. Red trail markers on the right tell you to bear right at the next fork in the road.

At 0.3 mile, you will finally reach the trail on your right. On your left is the outlet of Chub Pond that flows into Blue Mountain Lake. Shortly after the trail portion starts, you come to a log bridge crossing this stream and a fork in the trail. To your left is the south route to Castle Rock, while to your right is Upper Sargent Pond and the north route. Cross the bridge to follow the south route, a rolling trail through mixed hardwoods. Yellow disks emblazon the trail, and at 0.6 mile you can see Chub Pond and a broad wetland to your right. The view is limited, but better views of the pond are available on the return trip along the northern route. When I hiked the trail, rain had been falling sporadically for days, so the trail was very wet; in fact, it was basically a stream in some sections (particularly on the northern route). But judging by the number of mucky spots, it is safe to say that this trail is typically wet.

The trail is a deep-woods walk among tall hemlock, birch, maple, and spruce trees. The landscape is dotted with large, mossy boulders that hint at the large rock faces to come. At 0.8 mile you will

Castle Rock

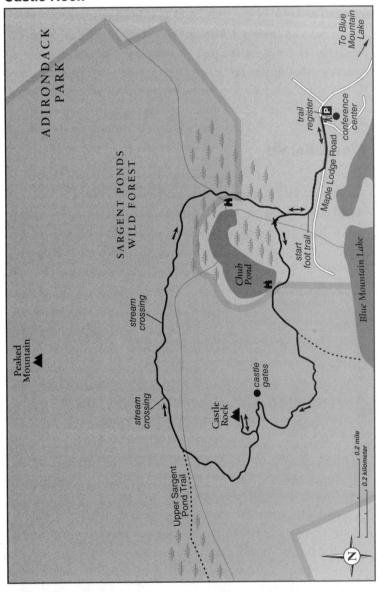

find a small dip, as well as a fork, in the trail; 0.3 mile to your left is Blue Mountain Lake, while Castle Rock is 0.7 mile to your right. After crossing a small brook, the trail begins to climb steadily. Openings in the forest canopy indicate that the lake sprawls off to your left, but you cannot see it until you reach the summit.

At 1.2 miles, you come to what I imagine to be the castle's gates. The base of the large granite outcrop towers above you on your right, with a narrow passage between it and some of the boulders that lie among the cliff's talus. Running water babbles underneath the sheer castle wall, sparking images of activities on the other side. Paths that eventually lead back to the main trail weave through the maze of boulders, providing opportunities for exploration.

Back along the trail, a brief climb brings you to the intersection of the northern route, on your left. The climb to Castle Rock's final lookout is on your right, through spruces and paper birches. You reach the summit as you squeeze through another narrow passage. Climbing atop the rock ledge on your left reveals views of the tree-covered mountains to the north. While this view is beautiful and panoramic, the real gem is the view from atop the ledge, or rather the southern turret, on your right. This sheer cliff 700 feet above Blue Mountain Lake provides vistas of the wooded islands that dot the lake. The cliff's

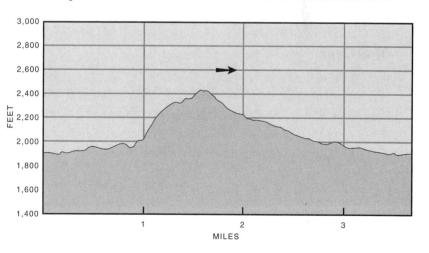

sheer walls and the way it juts out above the treeline evoke the feeling of being atop a lookout tower and, in combination with the "gate" at the base, give rise to the impression of a castle. Take caution around the cliff edge during wet or icy conditions.

Returning along the northern route, the trail is less steep and descends gradually with numerous stream crossings. This portion is marked with red Department of Environmental Conservation disks and is easy to follow. At 1.9 miles you cross a stream and come to a fork in the trail; the Upper Sargent Pond Trail heads off to your left, while to the right is the return to the trailhead and parking area. While the southern route definitely has some wet areas, the northern route has notably more and longer mucky spots. The forest matures as you descend, and you rock-hop across multiple streams that flow to your right. At 2.3 miles, you come to a meadow, where the sound of water rushing to your right is much more distinct. The trail flattens out a bit more, and the mucky areas become more frequent. You encounter Chub Pond again at 2.8 miles, with views of Castle Rock through the hemlocks that surround the wetland. Multiple vantage points of the pond are available along the trail, and shortly you come back to the juncture where the log bridge crosses the outlet of Chub Pond. The stroll back to the parking area passes quickly along the flat roads.

Directions

From the intersection of NY 28/NY 30/NY 28N in Blue Mountain Lake village, head north on NY 30/NY 28N. Turn left onto Maple Lodge Road at 0.6 mile. Continue on Maple Lodge Road 1.2 miles until you see the trail register, and park at the pulloff on the left side of the road before the Minnowbrook Conference Center.

22 Blue Ledges

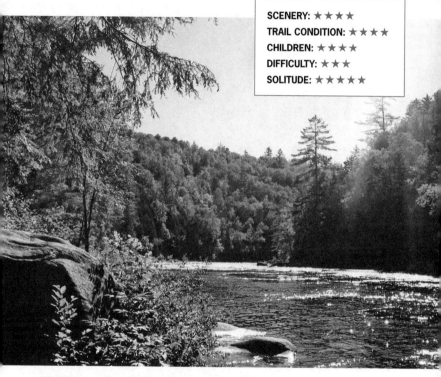

HUDSON RIVER DOWNSTREAM FROM BLUE LEDGES

GPS COORDINATES: N43° 49.957'   W74° 06.506'

DISTANCE & CONFIGURATION: 5.0-mile out-and-back

HIKING TIME: 2–3 hours

HIGHLIGHTS: Vertical cliffs in the Hudson River Gorge

ELEVATION: 1,592' at trailhead, 1,345' at lowest point

ACCESS: Open 24/7; no fees or permits required

MAPS: National Geographic *Adirondack Park, Northville/Raquette Lake* (#744)

FACILITIES: None

WHEELCHAIR ACCESS: No

CONTACTS: Siamese Ponds Wilderness: www.dec.ny.gov/lands/53172.html; Eastern Adirondack trail information: www.dec.ny.gov/outdoor/9199.html; emergency contact: 518-891-0235

Blue Ledges

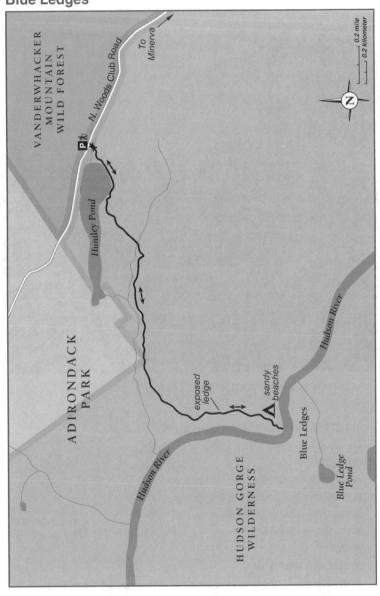

Overview

The beautiful stroll through a deep forest would be excuse enough to go on this hike, but the spectacular cliffs and sandy beaches in the Hudson River Gorge make it a must-do. In the height of summer, it's an excellent picnic or swimming destination, with the option for riverside camping. On dam-release days, especially during spring and fall, you will likely see rafters and kayakers navigating the turbulent rapids that flow at the base of these gigantic cliffs.

Route Details

The trail, marked with blue disks, begins across the road from the parking area on the left. Immediately cross a stream over a log-and-plank bridge, after which you'll find the trail register within a mucky area. The trail heads west toward the shore of Huntley Pond, where you have to pick your way through mud and tangles of roots. The walk along the shoreline requires a good deal of rock- and root-hopping to stay out of the muck, but this is very brief and followed by a slight climb into the hardwood forest.

At 0.5 mile pass between two large, moss-covered boulders, and then descend 0.3 mile to a stream. After crossing the stream, the

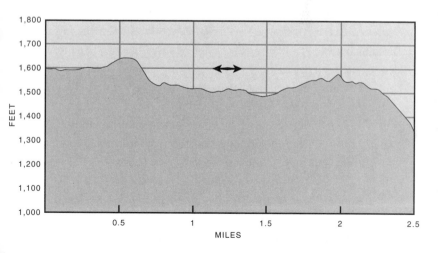

trail levels off, and it is easy going over the next 0.8 mile. The high canopy allows deep views into the forest on your left, while broad openings along the meandering stream to your right provide a stark contrast. You will likely notice some very large eastern white pines interspersed with birch and maple trees. At 1.5 miles you begin a 0.5-mile climb on the hill whose contour you have been following since the stream crossing. As you climb south, larger pine trees loom along the trail, and you will hear the Hudson's rushing waters to your right. Despite the thundering rapids that seem to be just beyond the treeline, you will not be able to see the river until you reach the trail's end. At 2 miles you cross a large, exposed portion of ledge that marks the beginning of the descent to the river. This lookout reveals nothing through the thick foliage of summer, but when the leaves fall, it promises excellent views. The last 0.5 mile of the trail is the steepest section but is easily managed on both the descent and the return climb. The eastern white pines sporadically encountered along the trail earlier now dominate the forest as you reach the riverbank.

You see glimpses of the ledges through the evergreen canopy, but the scale of the cliffs is not apparent until you reach the end of the trail. As you emerge directly on the riverbank, the Blue Ledges loom 300 feet high on the opposite shore.

The vertical wall of rock draped by pines and cedars, seen across the broad river, makes a dramatic and peaceful setting. Paths leading both up- and downriver explore the riverbank and take you to several sandy beaches. High water during spring and fall makes for whirlpools and rapids that are best observed or rafted with commercial outfitters. During periods of lower water in the summer, sheltered areas provide a good opportunity for swimming. If you choose to swim, be mindful that the river still has a powerful current and that dam releases from Lake Abanakee on Tuesdays, Thursdays, Saturdays, and Sundays raise the river by 2 feet. Upstream and around the bend is one major rapid, while downstream are some major Class IV and V rapids. These rapids are visible from the trail's end and provide a popular amusement shortly after midday on dam-release days. Designated riverside camping areas are also downstream near these treacherous rapids. You can reach the campsites by passing through a thicket of brush near the river's edge. Camping is limited to these areas, and they seem to fill up. Otherwise, Department of Environmental Conservation regulations require backpackers to set up camp at least 150 feet from any body of water. The Hudson River Gorge is an exceptionally beautiful destination in the Adirondacks, and unless you are willing to raft down the river, this trail is virtually the only way to see its beauty.

Directions

From the intersection of County Road 29/Main Street and NY 28N in Minerva, head 4.4 miles north on NY 28N, and turn left onto North Woods Club Road. The turn is more like bearing left, but it is located along a curve and hill, so you will likely miss it heading south along NY 28N, 11.7 miles south of the intersection of NY 28N and Blue Ridge Road in Newcomb. The dirt road is smooth and accessible for most vehicles. At 3.7 miles, you cross the Boreas River and see designated roadside camping on both sides of the road. The road climbs steeply afterward. As it descends, the trail sign is visible on the left at 6.7 miles. The parking area along North Woods Club Road could accommodate close to a dozen vehicles if parked close together and perpendicular to the road.

23

Hoffman Notch

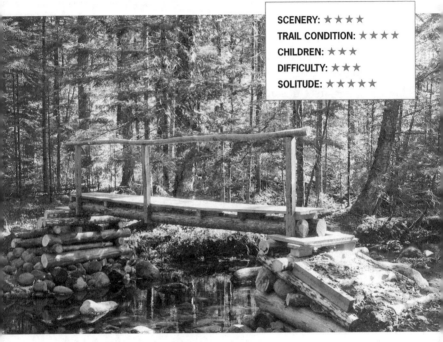

SCENERY: ★ ★ ★ ★
TRAIL CONDITION: ★ ★ ★ ★
CHILDREN: ★ ★ ★
DIFFICULTY: ★ ★ ★
SOLITUDE: ★ ★ ★ ★ ★

BRIDGE ACROSS HOFFMAN NOTCH BROOK

GPS COORDINATES: Southern trailhead: N43° 52.091'   W73° 53.338'
Northern trailhead: N43° 57.235'   W73° 50.196'

DISTANCE & CONFIGURATION: 7.5-mile point-to-point

HIKING TIME: 4–5 hours

HIGHLIGHTS: Isolated pond, streamside hiking

ELEVATION: 1,650' at trailhead, 1,190' at lowest point

ACCESS: Open 24/7; no fees or permits required

MAPS: Hoffman Notch Wilderness: tinyurl.com/hoffnotchmap; National Geographic *Adirondack Park, Lake George/Great Sacandaga* (#743)

FACILITIES: None

WHEELCHAIR ACCESS: No

CONTACTS: Hoffman Notch Wilderness: www.dec.ny.gov/lands/81598.html; Eastern Adirondack trail information: www.dec.ny.gov/outdoor/9199.html; emergency contact: 518-891-0235

Overview

Passing through this notch provides hikers with scenery and solitude. You follow a flat stream to a serene marsh, where Hoffman Mountain is framed in the background, and then down a fast-falling brook with innumerable small cascades. The trail is fairly easy, so fast and experienced hikers will find that they can traverse the notch in half the time, but this precludes enjoying the privacy along the picturesque trail.

Route Details

This point-to-point trail would be excellent in either direction but is probably easier and most enjoyable heading from south to north. Deciding which end to leave a car or where to be picked up all depends on circumstance, but it might be advisable to leave a car at the southern lot for extended trips. The southern lot is large and off the main road, while the northern end is probably easiest to give directions to. This would also be a great trip for the key-pass technique, where two parties start at opposite locations and exchange car keys when they pass each other, as no detours or side trips might cause them to miss each other. Directions here are given heading south to north.

The trail begins on the northwest corner of a large, grassy parking area off Loch Muller Road, which has ample space for dozens of cars. A 1-mile trail to Bailey Pond, on your left, is also located at the beginning of the Hoffman Notch Trail. Continue straight ahead on the abandoned road, marked in yellow for the entire trail, through the mixed hardwood forest. The wide, open road makes for easy travel, and you will quickly come within sight of the West Branch Trout Brook approximately 0.3 mile in. The trail heads west briefly, and you descend to a log-and-plank bridge. Like the numerous bridges near the end of the trail, the bridge has been handsomely built with substantial cribbing and stonework to bolster the crossing. Shortly after crossing the bridge, the road begins to transition into trail, but the going is still easy over the mostly rolling terrain.

Hoffman Notch

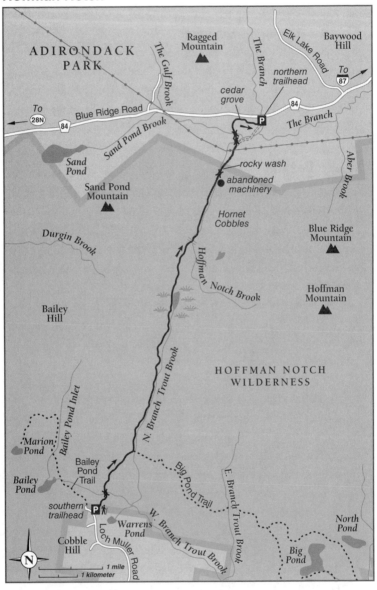

You will encounter a few seasonally muddy sections before reaching the only other trail intersection at 1.3 miles. The main trail continues straight ahead following yellow disks, while the trail to the right is marked in blue and leads to another access point along Hoffman Road. If you seek an extended trip, you can add almost 6 miles by starting at Hoffman Road. The North Branch Trout Brook begins to flow on your right after you pass this intersection and accompanies you all the way to Big Marsh at the halfway point. Approximately 2 miles in, you pass an enormous erratic alongside the trail. Though many may think I am an erratic on the trail, talking into the voice recorder dangling from the front of my pack, erratics are actually large boulders that were deposited by receding glaciers. They are termed *erratic* because they typically do not fit in with the surrounding landscape, due to either their composition or, more likely, their location. The trail winds to and from the banks of the brook numerous times, and at 2.3 miles, it passes nearly through the water as it cuts its way north along the mossy banks. The brook flows over mostly flat terrain and consequently is very slow moving, especially when you reach the beaver dam at 2.5 miles. Evergreens dot the banks along this section, and you will notice that the terrain grows ever steeper on your left as you head toward the midpoint of the notch. Here, the notch

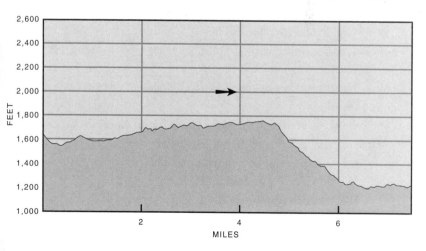

is the low point between the Washburn Ridge on your left and the Texas Ridge on your right. Roughly 0.5 mile ahead, the marshland truly begins, with grassy islands interspersed along the brook as it meanders wider near the notch's peak. The marshlands create broad, open sections in the forest, and soon Hoffman Mountain begins to loom across the scenic wetlands. At 3.5 miles the trail descends briefly to the wide, open waters of the marsh—though *lake* or *pond* would likely be a more apt description. A few skeletal trees remain in the open waters, enhancing the wild character of this remote area.

Numerous vantage points for scenic photos are found all along the trail as it winds along the hemlock- and birch-lined western shore. You leave Big Marsh's shores at 4 miles, but the trail continues along flat terrain through mixed hardwoods another 0.8 mile. A small, seasonal brook joins you on your left, and shortly after it, you reach Hoffman Notch Brook, which tumbles in at a small cascade on your right and forms a deep pool that can be passed across a worn tree. Rock-hopping might be a better option in wet conditions, as the tree is nearly worn smooth.

The trail continues on the opposite shore under a thick canopy of hardwoods, and several wet sections turn the trail into a mire at points. At this point the brook is descending rapidly, forming innumerable cascades with a low rumbling that drowns out most other forest sounds. The trail parallels the brook on an elevated ridge along the eastern banks approximately 0.3 mile before descending to the rock- and boulder-strewn brook at 5.1 miles, where you cross to the western bank. Trail markers are absent or difficult to follow in this section, but if you keep the brook in sight and look for the worn path, you can easily find your way to the crossing and the yellow trail markers. The waters are falling rapidly at this point, but the boulders are so large that it's easy to hop across the brook to the opposite shore, where the trail continues to descend on the western bank.

The notch is very distinct along this portion of the trail, as you pass the several sheer rock faces of Washburn Ridge on your left and the terrain, Hornet Cobbles, grows steeper on the right. Roughly

5.8 miles in, the trail transitions into an abandoned road with built-up banks, and the hiking gets easier. At 6 miles you pass a rusted piece of abandoned track machinery on your right that reminds you of the persistent regenerative power of nature.

At 6.1 miles you reach a rocky wash where a low bridge spans Hoffman Notch Brook. This crossing marks the end of the descent, and it is mostly rolling terrain for the next 1.4 miles to the northern terminus. At 6.5 miles you pass through a clearing where power lines have cut a swath through the wilderness; shortly after, you reach another sturdy bridge that re-crosses Hoffman Notch Brook. This flat section of the trail is a rerouting of the often-flooded north end and crosses a couple more bridges. The trail swings east through a notable stand of cedars and then intersects the old north road at 7.4 miles. The rusted front end of a classic car is found at this junction, only a few hundred yards from the trail terminus at Blue Ridge Road.

Directions

SOUTHERN TRAILHEAD   From I-87, take Exit 28, and head east on NY 74. Immediately turn right onto US 9 in Schroon Lake. In 2.9 miles, turn right onto County Road 24/Hoffman Road. In 5.4 miles, turn right onto Potash Hill Road. At 1.1 miles turn right onto Lock Muller Road. Follow Lock Muller Road 1.3 miles, and look for a gravel drive on the right. Follow the gravel drive a short way to the large, grassy parking area.

NORTHERN TRAILHEAD   From I-87, take Exit 29 (Newcomb/North Hudson). Head west on CR 84/Blue Ridge Road and go 5.5 miles. The parking area is a small gravel drive on the left.

Eastern (Hikes 24–29)

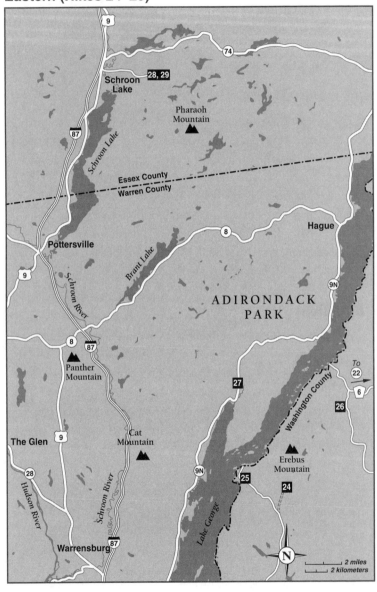

9

74

Schroon Lake 28, 29

Pharaoh Mountain

87

Schroon Lake

Essex County

Warren County

8

Hague

Pottersville

9

Brant Lake

Schroon River

9N

A D I R O N D A C K
P A R K

8 87

Panther Mountain

27

To 22

6

The Glen 9

Cat Mountain

26

Washington County

Hudson River

Schroon River

9N

Erebus Mountain

28

25

24

Warrensburg 87

Lake George

N

2 miles
2 kilometers

Eastern

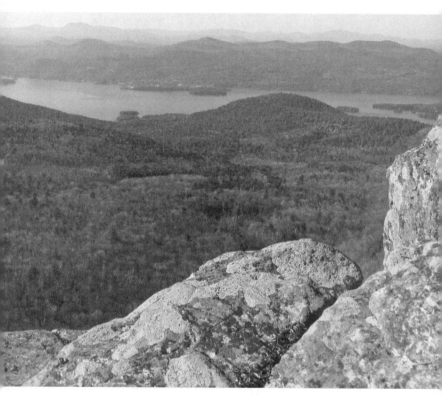

LAKE GEORGE SEEN FROM SLEEPING BEAUTY MOUNTAIN (*Trail 24, Sleeping Beauty Mountain, page 166*)

24 Sleeping Beauty Mountain

SCENERY: ★ ★ ★ ★
TRAIL CONDITION: ★ ★ ★ ★ ★
CHILDREN: ★ ★ ★ ★ ★
DIFFICULTY: ★ ★ ★
SOLITUDE: ★ ★

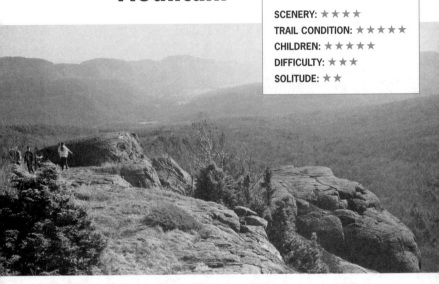

VIEW OF LOWER LOOKOUT FROM UPPER LOOKOUT

GPS COORDINATES: N43° 32.971'   W73° 33.369'

DISTANCE & CONFIGURATION: 3.3-mile out-and-back from Dacy Clearing (seasonal access) or 6.5-mile out-and-back from Hog Town parking area

HIKING TIME: 2–3 hours

HIGHLIGHTS: Sheer cliffs, panoramic views

ELEVATION: 1,335' at trailhead, 2,347' at highest point

ACCESS: Open 24/7; no fees or permits required. Access along Shelving Rock Road is seasonal and subject to town of Fort Ann approval. Dacy Clearing Road is not plowed and is closed during mud season (early spring).

MAPS: National Geographic *Adirondack Park, Lake George/Great Sacandaga* (#743)

FACILITIES: Picnic tables, pit toilets

WHEELCHAIR ACCESS: No

COMMENTS: Timber rattlesnakes are known to occupy the shores of Lake George, so be cautious when stepping over logs. Read more about timber rattlesnakes in the section on Animal, Insect, and Plant Hazards (page 20).

CONTACTS: Eastern Adirondack trail information: www.dec.ny.gov/outdoor/9199.html; emergency contact: 518-891-0235

Overview

The sheer cliffs are a spectacle in and of themselves, but once you add the views of Lake George from Sleeping Beauty's summit, this becomes a must-visit trail. Though the hike is steep in sections, the short distance from Dacy Clearing places it easily within the grasp of hikers of all experience levels. A longer approach or additional circuit can be added for hikers who desire a more extensive adventure.

Route Details

To reach the trailhead at Dacy Clearing, you can either drive or hike 1.6 miles from the Hog Town parking area. The road, though a bit narrow, is in good shape, and vehicles in good condition should have no difficulty reaching the clearing. This way passes multiple campsites, historic sites, and additional trailheads, so hikers wishing for additional interest or mileage may want to consider starting from the Hog Town parking area.

Dacy Clearing has a large parking area, as well as some day-use facilities, including picnic tables and pit toilets, so don't be surprised to find many people who choose this as a destination in itself. The trailhead is in the southern corner of the parking area, just to the side of a vehicle barrier and stream. Yellow disks mark this portion of the trail. The trail heads south but almost immediately switches back north and begins a steady climb. The trail register is a few hundred yards from the switchback, and when you see how full it is, it is obvious that this is a popular trail. The trail, wide enough for two to hike side by side, was once a part of the Knapp Estate's road network that weaves through the area. In 1931, 4,300 acres of the Knapp Estate were acquired by the state, including much of the southeastern section of Lake George Wild Forest.

Less than 0.5 mile in, the trail switches back southeast, and the climb slackens a bit. During the height of summer, the dense canopy masks the sheer cliffs of Sleeping Beauty, but in the fall or winter, the cliffs are more visible and soon loom ahead of you. A

Sleeping Beauty Mountain

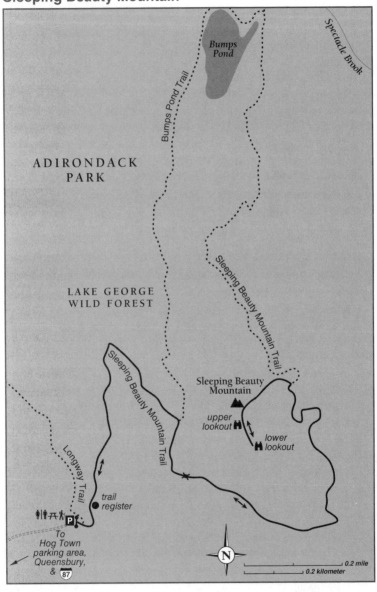

Bumps Pond

Spectacle Brook

Bumps Pond Trail

ADIRONDACK
PARK

LAKE GEORGE
WILD FOREST

Sleeping Beauty Mountain Trail

Sleeping Beauty Mountain Trail

Sleeping Beauty
Mountain

upper
lookout

lower
lookout

Longway Trail

trail
register

To
Hog Town
parking area,
Queensbury,
& 87

N

0.2 mile

0.2 kilometer

large, angular boulder at 0.6 mile marks a T in the trail, and the magnitude of the cliffs becomes apparent even with leafed-out trees. The trail to the left, marked in yellow, leads to Bumps Pond as well as a circuit trail that returns to Sleeping Beauty Summit. The alternate route is more than 2 miles to the summit, while to the right, the distance to the summit is a little over a mile. To the right, marked with blue disks, is a more direct and, in my opinion, more impressive route to the summit because you hike along the base of the cliffs.

The trail to the right leaves the old road network behind, and you traverse a narrow foot trail through a tiny hemlock grove. For the next 0.4 mile, you will be hiking along a flat plateau on the south side of the mountain, with truly impressive views of the sheer cliff and the tumble of boulders at its base. Through the surrounding canopy, you can catch brief glimpses of the mountains to the southwest, but they don't compare to the vistas at the summit. The grade is basically flat, and though there are a few wet spots, it is easy going. At 0.8 mile, you cross a 10-foot bridge, and the trail swings east. The trail dips down briefly, but at 1 mile you begin the climb to the summit. Multiple switchbacks make the climb easier, and at 1.1 miles, you make your way up a substantially built-up switchback with a high rock wall.

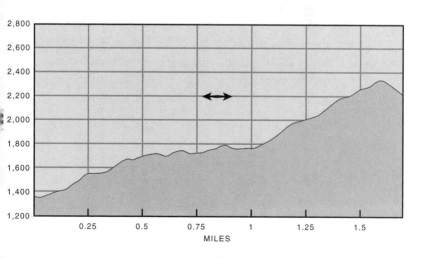

After this point, the trail weaves its way north on the east side of the cliffs, and views disappear as the forest becomes more coniferous. At 1.6 miles, you reach a Y in the trail. To the right is the trail to Bumps Pond and the circuit mentioned previously, while straight ahead is the summit, 0.1 mile. When you reach the end of the trail, you can view the panorama that opens out before you from several open ledges. Immediately in front of you is a large outcrop where people congregate; a higher but smaller outcrop is also to your right and slightly behind you, and a large, lower one is to the south. At the lower lookout, you have the advantage of seeing your path along the base of the cliffs. Expansive views to the west, south, and north show various portions of Lake George and the surrounding mountains from all of these lookouts, and there is plenty of room to sit and enjoy the views. Return the way you came for a total trip length of 3.3 miles, or take the circuit for a total length of 4.4 miles.

Directions

From the intersection of US 9 and NY 149 in Queensbury, south of Lake George and north of Glens Falls, head east along NY 149. Turn left onto Buttermilk Falls Road at 6 miles. Keep left at 3.1 miles where Buttermilk Falls Road turns into Sly Pond Road. Sly Pond Road turns into Shelving Rock Road at 5.7 miles, just past the intersection with Hog Town Road on the right. Continue on Shelving Rock Road 0.8 mile to the Hog Town parking area. Park here if you desire a longer trip. Otherwise, continue down the one-lane road 1.6 miles to Dacy Clearing.

Shelving Rock Falls

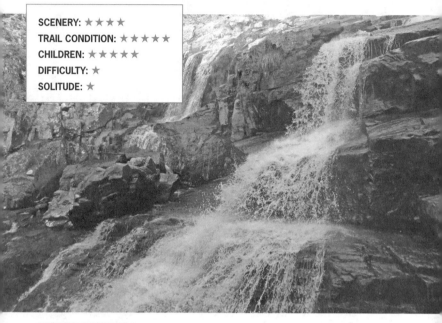

SHELVING ROCK FALLS

GPS COORDINATES: N43° 33.357'   W73° 36.184'

DISTANCE & CONFIGURATION: 1.5-mile out-and-back to falls, 4.1-mile loop along lake

HIKING TIME: 2 hours

HIGHLIGHTS: Spectacular waterfall, lakeside hiking, old foundation

ELEVATION: 450' at trailhead, with no significant rise along trail

ACCESS: Open 24/7; no fees or permits required; access along Shelving Rock Road is seasonal and subject to town of Fort Ann approval

MAPS: National Geographic *Adirondack Park, Lake George/Great Sacandaga* (#743)

FACILITIES: None

WHEELCHAIR ACCESS: No

COMMENTS: Timber rattlesnakes are known to occupy the shores of Lake George, so be cautious when stepping over logs. Read more about timber rattlesnakes in the section on Animal, Insect, and Plant Hazards (page 20).

CONTACTS: Eastern Adirondack trail information: www.dec.ny.gov/outdoor/9199.html; emergency contact: 518-891-0235

Shelving Rock Falls

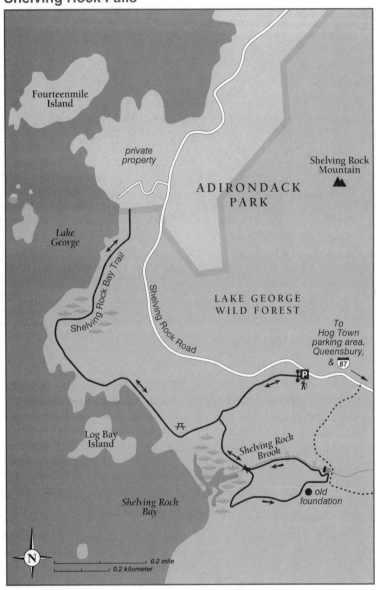

Overview

Following the shore of Lake George, the trail system around Shelving Rock Falls was once carriage roads and therefore makes for some of the easiest hiking in the Adirondacks. Though the trails are easy, they are beautiful and offer an array of scenery and history. You can explore the trails and destinations in a variety of ways, so consider the system of trails more of a destination than simply a hike.

Route Details

Though many smaller parking areas are along Shelving Rock Road, the spaces are very limited, often with room for only one or two cars, and not clearly marked as parking areas. Because the entire roadside is plastered with signs warning that cars parked along the road will be ticketed or towed, I would not plan on finding parking except in the large parking area for which the signs are obvious and directions are given. Likewise, trails leading to Lake George's shores are not clearly marked at the other parking areas, while the trail from the main parking area is impossible to miss.

On the right side of the parking area, walk past the vehicle barrier and down the broad access road. You have probably noticed

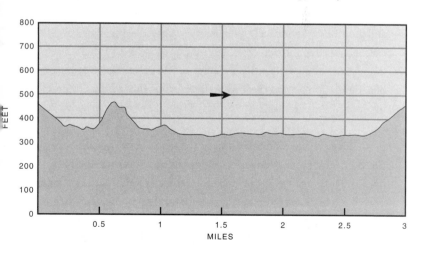

that there is no trail register, nor are there any trail markers, but it is practically impossible to lose your way. Likewise, Shelving Rock Road and Lake George border the trail system, so you cannot wander far off the trail before regaining your bearings. Less than 0.3 mile in, you will come to a fork in the trail. Straight ahead is the main portion of the lakeside trails, while to your left are the falls. Continue to the left, and cross Shelving Rock Brook over a wooden bridge at 0.4 mile. On the opposite side of the bridge, you may notice a footpath to your left. This footpath can be used to climb to—or as your return route from—the falls. The stroll along the designated trail is an easier approach and has its own charms near the top.

You may have noticed that the trail system is more like a network of roads. Indeed, this area of Lake George Wild Forest was once a part of the Knapp Estate, and the trails were formerly carriage roads. The extensive work employed to level the terrain and build these roads becomes evident when you pass a large rock retaining wall on your left. The wall is part of a switchback that leads up the hill that eventually climbs to the top of Shelving Rock Falls. Tall pines thoroughly shade the area, and as you reach the height of the climb, you will notice a lone-wolf pine on your right.

Lone-wolf trees are trees that grow in open fields and eventually get overtopped when the forest takes over the field. Often short and gnarly, they eventually get shaded out and die, but they become excellent shelter and den trees. Any doubts that the environment has undergone a major transition are removed when you see the remains of a foundation behind the lone-wolf pine. This ruin adds an interesting spot for exploration, but the roar of the falls ahead will likely keep you from dallying long.

The carriage road takes you to the dam above the falls. Off to the right, the carriage road continues back to Shelving Rock Road, but straight ahead you can make out the caissons that once supported a bridge over the artificial wetland that sprawls out before you. Across the dam, you can see a trail and might be tempted to cross the top of the dam, but do not attempt it. Bear in mind that

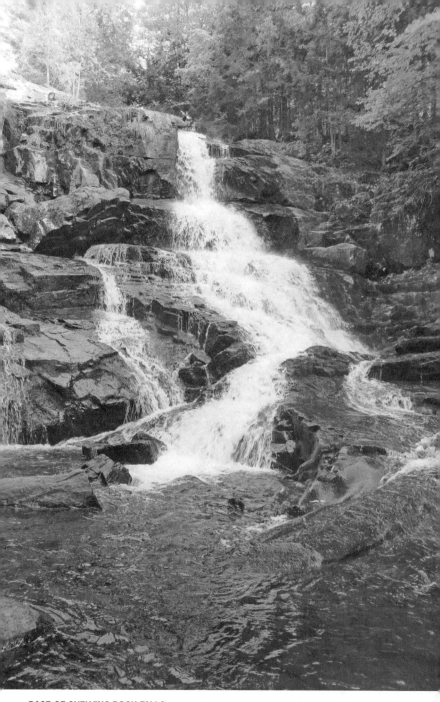

BASE OF SHELVING ROCK FALLS

the dam is narrow and covered in slick algae, and many people have been injured or have died here. The best and, coincidentally, most scenic way to reach the other side is at the base of the falls.

A short scramble downhill will take you there. Keep an eye out for a protruding rock on the right that makes an outstanding point from which to view and photograph the falls. The falls cascade 70–80 feet through and over large protrusions of ledge, with a deep pool beneath. You can return along the carriage road or take the more interesting footpath down beside Shelving Rock Brook. Besides adding a little more interest to the hike, this path has the benefit of revealing another smaller falls about midway down to the bridge previously crossed. You will have to scramble along rocks and roots to get down, but the trail is no different from typical Adirondack trails.

Back on the trail, you have the option to head back to your vehicle, but it would be a shame to miss the walk along Lake George that awaits you by continuing to your left at the first fork. The trail along the lakeshore is level, passes within feet of the lake for long portions, and has a few excellent lookouts. The trail ends at private property, and you can return to the parking lot along Shelving Rock Road, but the trail along the lake is so pleasant that it is by far your better option.

Directions

From the intersection of US 9 and NY 149 in Queensbury, south of Lake George and north of Glens Falls, head east along NY 149. Turn left onto Buttermilk Falls Road at 6 miles. Keep left at 3.1 miles, where Buttermilk Falls Road turns into Sly Pond Road. Sly Pond Road turns into Shelving Rock Road at 5.7 miles, just past the intersection with Hog Town Road on the right. Continue on Shelving Rock Road 1.8 miles, where you pass the parking area for primitive campsites and register for the area. Continue to the left on Shelving Rock Road another 1.8 miles to the parking area on your left. This is the second parking area on the south side of the road, past the Shelving Rock Mountain parking area on the north side of the road.

Black Mountain

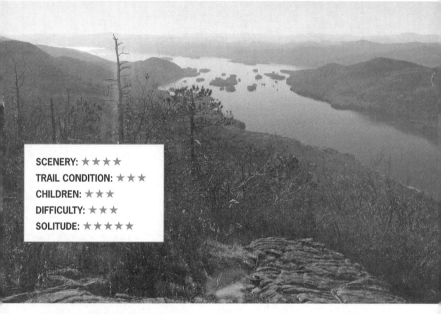

26

SCENERY: ★ ★ ★ ★
TRAIL CONDITION: ★ ★ ★
CHILDREN: ★ ★ ★
DIFFICULTY: ★ ★ ★
SOLITUDE: ★ ★ ★ ★ ★

LOOKING SOUTH AT LAKE GEORGE

GPS COORDINATES: N43° 36.702'   W73° 29.612'

DISTANCE & CONFIGURATION: 6.7-mile balloon

HIKING TIME: 4–5 hours

HIGHLIGHTS: Panoramic views, remote ponds, beaver activity, lake views

ELEVATION: 1,564' at trailhead, 2,646' at Black Mountain peak

ACCESS: Open 24/7; no fees or permits required

MAPS: National Geographic *Adirondack Park, Lake George/Great Sacandaga* (#743)

FACILITIES: None

WHEELCHAIR ACCESS: No

COMMENTS: Timber rattlesnakes are known to occupy the shores of Lake George, so be cautious when stepping over logs. Read more about timber rattlesnakes in the section on Animal, Insect, and Plant Hazards (page 20).

CONTACTS: Eastern Adirondack trail information: www.dec.ny.gov/outdoor/9199.html; emergency contact: 518-891-0235

Black Mountain

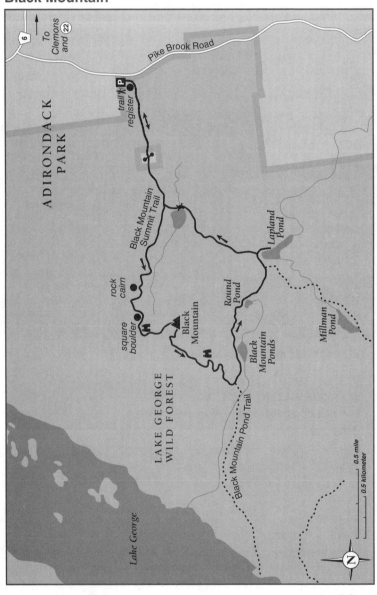

Overview

Black Mountain is the highest peak in the southeastern Adirondack–Lake George region. It lies a little farther from the bustling heart of Lake George, so hikers seeking more solitude in the eastern Adirondacks may find this an excellent choice. By summiting from the north and descending along the southern slope, you will traverse a wide variety of environs and maximize the number of panoramic views.

Route Details

The parking area off Pike Brook Road is sufficient for roughly a dozen cars conscientiously parked. The trailhead and trail register are on the western edge of the pulloff. The initial section of the trail, marked in red, follows a gravel access road that almost immediately turns sharply left and climbs steadily up and away from the parking area. After swinging west, the road levels off and continues 0.6 mile to where a building with a metal roof comes into view. A vehicle barrier blocks the road, and the trail—indicated by a brown trail sign—diverges to the right into the forest along a more traditional footpath.

The trail continues a little more than 0.3 mile along flat terrain among maple and beech trees to a trail intersection, 1 mile overall.

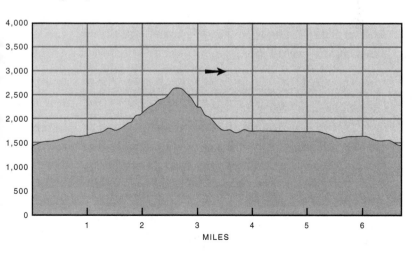

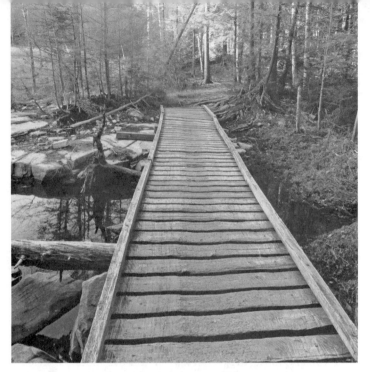

A BRIDGE ALONG THE TRAIL KEEPS YOUR FEET DRY AT THIS CROSSING.

To the left (south) are the remote ponds and return leg of the trip. Continue straight, and you soon have to hop across a small stream, after which you continue west along a fairly gentle grade. About 0.5 mile past the intersection, the trail is bisected by another seasonal stream that spills into a stream flowing to the left. Shortly after rock-hopping across the seasonal stream, the trail takes a sharp turn right (north). It parallels the stream briefly north, swings west, and then becomes steeper once it heads west again, briefly paralleling and running through the seasonal stream as it climbs.

After crossing and leaving the streambed, you will pass a rock cairn on the left, 1.9 miles from the start. Shortly after, the trail swings west and the climbing continues to steepen. Spruce and birch trees dominate the forest along with verdant, moss-covered rocks. The primeval and dark setting of the northern, shaded side of the mountain is in stark contrast to the brighter deciduous, southern slope found on the return leg. This dark setting is even more dominant as the trail swings nearly south. Along a brief level section of trail, you pass by a large, square boulder to the left, just before a fork in the trail, 2.5 miles overall.

The left fork is a lightly worn path, while the right fork is a more heavily worn, cobble-strewn trail that leads to the summit. Bear right and head uphill to where the trail swings sharply north as you make the final ascent. The inaccessible fire tower and a windmill soon come into view as you make the final approach along an exposed ledge. Just before heading up to the peak and its amalgam of technology, check out the small lookout on the right near a memorial placard nailed to a tree. At the peak, there are limited places to stop and take in the view, so on busy or windy days this lookout may be the more desirable place to take a break.

On top of the summit are a windmill, a power transfer station, solar panels, fencing, and a fire tower, all dedicated to emergency communications. They occupy most of the summit, and there are not many places that would be considered a good place to rest. The one exception is atop a rock outcrop on the northern tip of the peak, just behind the fire tower. To reach this spot, head between the windmill and fence to where a trail sign indicates the direction to the return trip, and head right. A large rock partially shields you from the incongruous pieces of civilization, and great panoramic views of the northern tip of Lake George sprawl out before you.

To return, you could head back the way you came, but you would miss some of the great views of southern Lake George and wildly different ecosystems encountered along the northern pond route. Head back to the trail sign, and proceed southeast in the direction of Black Mountain Pond Trail junction.

As you begin the descent (roughly 900 feet over the next mile), the trail takes on a very different character. Instead of the boreal and wet setting of the northern slope, the southern slope is dry and grassy with a canopy of deciduous trees, most notably oaks farther down the mountain. It's a stark contrast but also the perfect setting for timber rattlesnakes that like to bask in the sun on open ledges, so be mindful when stepping over logs and rocks. The open ledges are also the best spots to take in the panoramic views of Lake George available at several locations along the steep descent. Access the first lookout by following one of several herd paths through the surrounding scrub, about 0.1 mile down. Because of the aforementioned snakes, this might not be the best for those who are squeamish. The second lookout is along a ledge near a large boulder beside the trail, about 0.25 mile farther along the descent; it requires a small amount of navigating off trail. Don't worry if you don't want to bushwhack to these lookouts because another splendid one is found 0.3 mile farther.

The third lookout, located at 3.3 miles overall, is a broad opening along the trail with a beautiful view of the southern portion of Lake George; you reach it just after a large switchback that leads beneath a steep wall of rock. One final lookout of note is a little less than 0.1 mile ahead. This one is just to the left before another switchback swings the trail west. The open, grassy ledge is nestled among tall oaks and provides a view of not only Lake George but also the pristine ponds found farther along the trail. This is the last of the great viewing areas along the descent, which continues along many switchbacks another 0.25 mile and 200 feet to where the trail levels off and soon swings east.

At 3.6 miles reach the Black Mountain Pond Trail junction to the right and the return to Pike Brook Road via Black Mountain Pond straight ahead. Continue straight, now following blue trail markers, less than 0.25 mile to where Black Mountain Pond comes into view. Once up and over a small knoll, the dark pond and a grassy marsh sprawl out before you. Nearby you traverse an open ledge that dives into the water; the Black Mountain Pond Lean-To sits just uphill from this ledge. The trail continues to skirt the pond's edge briefly before veering off into the surrounding forest. As you leave the pond behind, pass through a long, wet area, and then reach a stream crossing, 4.2 miles. This is the beginning of the long, sinuous wetland that feeds Round Pond. Once across this feeder brook, bear right and follow the wetland to the cattail-lined pond. The trail weaves along the shore, often within inches of the high water, along sections where the cattails are so thick and close that they form a veritable wall.

As the trail heads away from Round Pond, a mossy swamp flanks the trail to the right and shortly reaches another trail intersection, 4.6 miles overall. To the right are Millman and Fishbrook Ponds, while to the left is the trail back to Pike Brook Road. Turn left (north) following yellow trail markers, and quickly reach one more intersection. To the right (south) is the 0.1-mile-long trail that leads to the Lapland Pond Lean-To. The left fork, straight, leads north to Pike Brook Road.

Continue north roughly a mile to reach the first trail junction and end of the loop portion of the hike. Initially all along this northward trek, the sections of the trail weave in and out of a streambed and include some long, muddy portions. About halfway to the junction, you will have to rock-hop across a rocky brook that bisects the trail. As you near the intersection, the trail dips down toward a wide, marshy area with a beaver dam. At the tip of this marsh, you reach a heavy timber-and-log bridge that crosses the marsh's outlet, 0.2 mile shy of the junction ahead. Once you reach the junction, turn right and follow the path previously trodden 1 mile to Pike Brook Road for an overall trip length of 6.7 miles.

Directions

FROM THE SOUTH   From the intersection of US 4 and NY 22 in Whitehall, continue north 7.1 miles along NY 22, and turn left onto County Road 6. After 2.6 miles turn left onto Pike Brook Road. After 0.8 mile the parking area will be on the right.

FROM THE NORTH   From the intersection of NY 9N and NY 22 in Ticonderoga, head southeast 19.2 miles along NY 22 S/NY 74 E. Turn right onto CR 6. After 2.6 miles turn left onto Pike Brook Road. After 0.8 mile the parking area will be on the right.

Tongue Mountain Range

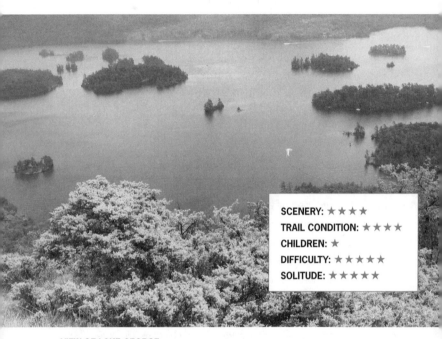

VIEW OF LAKE GEORGE

GPS COORDINATES: N43° 37.767'   W73° 36.489'

DISTANCE & CONFIGURATION: 12.6-mile loop (side trips not included)

HIKING TIME: 8–10 hours

HIGHLIGHTS: Multiple peaks with panoramic views, lakeside hiking, waterfall

ELEVATION: 403' at trailhead, 1,725' at highest point

ACCESS: Open 24/7; no fees or permits required

MAPS: National Geographic *Adirondack Park, Lake George/Great Sacandaga* (#743)

FACILITIES: None

WHEELCHAIR ACCESS: No

COMMENTS: Timber rattlesnakes are known to occupy the shores of Lake George, so be cautious when stepping over logs. Read more about timber rattlesnakes in the section on Animal, Insect, and Plant Hazards (page 20).

CONTACTS: Eastern Adirondack trail information: www.dec.ny.gov/outdoor/9199.html; emergency contact: 518-891-0235

Overview

There are multiple ways to explore the Tongue Mountain Range, but this loop combines some of the best features into an extended day hike. Multiple peaks offer innumerable panoramic views of Lake George, as well as some pleasant hiking along old Civilian Conservation Corps (CCC) horse trails following the lakeshore. Along the ridgeline, there are few sources of water, so bring your own supply to drink.

Route Details

Timber rattlesnakes are one of the few venomous species of snakes found in New York and are seldom seen, even in areas where they are known to live. The Tongue Mountain Range, as well as other areas along Lake George, is one of these few places and, though it is unlikely that you will encounter one, it is advisable to take precautions. See the section on animal hazards, page 20, and educate anyone unfamiliar with snakes. The simplest ways to avoid a mishap are to look where you step and to give the snake plenty of room should you see one.

The trailhead is a short distance south of the parking area along NY 9N. Turn left onto the trail, marked in red, and you will find the trail register several hundred yards ahead. The trail descends through a stand of pines, and you pass what looks to be a fork on your left but is actually just a short footpath. Continue to your right downhill, and soon reach a boardwalk that crosses the marsh surrounding Northwest Bay Brook. You reach a fork in the trail at 0.4 mile. To your right is the return leg of your trip along the Northwest Bay of Lake George, marked in blue. Continue straight, along the red-marked trail, which soon begins its ascent to the ridgeline. You will hear a waterfall off to your right shortly after the intersection. To view the 20-foot-high cascade, follow the barely discernible path on your right, or let the sounds of the falls guide you to the steep banks overlooking them.

The trail continues to climb, and you will cross and recross the seasonal stream that leads to the waterfall over log-and-plank bridges. The pitch has steadily increased, and soon steep ledges loom

Tongue Mountain Range

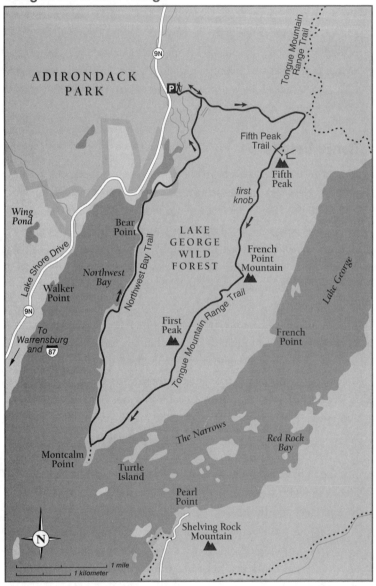

ADIRONDACK
PARK

9N

P

Tongue Mountain Range Trail

Fifth Peak Trail

Fifth Peak

first knob

Wing Pond

Bear Point

LAKE GEORGE WILD FOREST

French Point Mountain

Lake George

Lake Shore Drive

Northwest Bay Trail

Northwest Bay

Walker Point

9N

French Point

To Warrensburg and 87

First Peak

Tongue Mountain Range Trail

The Narrows

Red Rock Bay

Montcalm Point

Turtle Island

Pearl Point

Shelving Rock Mountain

N

1 mile

1 kilometer

on your left. After walking in the shadow of these ledges, you make a final ascent over a built-up switchback to a brief plateau, a little less than 1 mile from the start. The approximate 0.3-mile stroll along the hemlock-shrouded plateau is a welcome break from the ascent, but you soon begin to climb again along a switchback. After more marshy areas and a little more climbing, you soon reach a four-way intersection at 2 miles. To your left, marked in blue, is the ridge trail north to Five Mile Mountain, Deer Leap, and the northern trailhead along NY 9N. Straight ahead, marked in red, is the trail down to Five Mile Point on the shores of Lake George. Follow the blue-marked trail south, to your right, toward Fifth Peak, French Point Mountain, and Montcalm Point along Lake George. The trip south is a bit like a roller coaster as you navigate up and down the numerous peaks and valleys that make up the dragon spine–like ridge.

The trail climbs the next 0.4 mile to where you reach the intersection with Fifth Peak Trail, marked in yellow. The summit is 0.3 mile along this spur. A lean-to is also located along this trail for those wishing to make it an overnight trip. There is no water, so campers should plan accordingly, as it is a steep climb to the lakeshore or any other source of water.

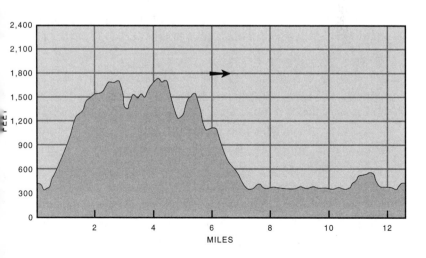

The trail continues straight, still marked in blue, around the west side of the mountain along a fairly level section. Views of the main portion of Lake George to the east are shortly followed with a view straight down to the Northwest Bay. The trail descends steeply after this point, and the roller coaster/sawtooth portion of the trail begins in earnest. After descending roughly 350 feet in less than 0.3 mile, you immediately begin to climb again to an unnamed knob, 3.6 miles at its top. This begins a series of steep ascents to fine views of the lake, followed by sharp descents. Each tiny summit provides a great place to stop, but if you plan on making only one stop along your traverse, I recommend waiting until you reach French Point Mountain, roughly 0.8 mile ahead after this first major descent. You scramble up, over, and down yet another knob, 4 miles, before you begin the final climb to French Point Mountain, 4.3 miles and 1,756 feet of elevation. If you haven't taken in the beauty of the roughly 200 verdant islands dotting the deep blue of Lake George, now is surely the time. The steep eastern side of the range has been swept with fire numerous times, and only scrubby trees dot the slope down to the lake, so panoramic views, open fields, and ledges are the norm and provide innumerable spots to stop.

You weave up and down another tiny knob before seeing First Peak looming to the south. This peak is the last major dip and climb of the dragon's spine before the trail makes its last descent to Lake George at Montcalm Point. The trail descends approximately 500 feet before climbing another 300 feet over the next 1.4 miles on your way to First Peak, 5.7 miles from the start. Breathtaking views await you here, as well as along the majority of the descent to the lake. You are a little less than halfway through the hike, though you will have probably spent more than half of your planned time along the trail. Not to worry—the trail is mostly downhill or level as you complete the loop. Views of the Lake George Narrows sprawl out before you as you descend the mostly exposed portion of the tongue. Mileage to the innumerable vantage points would probably provide more confusion than any measure of progress. However, you reach the final knob approximately 0.5 mile

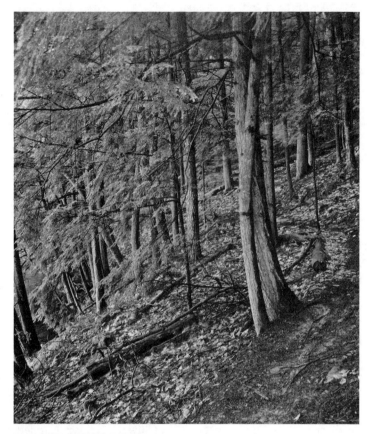

TRAIL BESIDE NORTHWEST BAY

after First Peak and, shortly after, delve back into the deeper woods. You reach the final intersection along the trail, 7.6 miles, at a wide and mucky area. To the left is Montcalm Point, 0.2 mile, a welcome respite along the shores. Though the side trip is definitely worth a visit, those pressed for time can rest assured that numerous sections along the return trip come within feet of the lake and provide points to stop and soak your feet or even take a swim.

To return, continue straight/right along the blue-marked trail north. Shortly after the intersection, the trail passes within feet of the lake but soon arcs east into the forest to bypass a small section of private land. After this brief diversion, you rejoin the lakeshore and find that the trail generally follows the lake. The farther north you go, the better the condition of the trail and the easier the path. You pass several openings along the lake, along with stream crossings, abandoned fire pits, and swimming holes, so if time permits, enjoy the numerous points of interest, or plan to take a late-hike rest.

Former CCC work is evident all along this return portion as you pass built-up crossings, rock walls, and other trail developments that make this portion of the trail truly a pleasure. At 10.6 miles, you reach the marsh where Northwest Bay Brook meets its namesake bay. It is only 1.6 miles back to the intersection and 2 miles to the parking area. An occasional passing truck along NY 9N will remind you of this proximity, though the trail heads northeast into the forest a bit, and roadside noise is mostly drowned out. The trail climbs slightly during this 0.8-mile arc into the forest and soon descends back toward the marsh. Soon after the descent, you reach the trail intersection at 12.2 miles. Continue left back to your vehicle at the quarry-side parking area for a total trip of 12.6 miles (not including side trips).

Directions

From I-87, take Exit 24 (County Road 11/Bolton Landing/Riverbank Road), and head 4.7 miles east on CR 11/Riverbank Road. Turn left onto NY 9N/Lake Shore Drive, and head northeast 4.5 miles. The parking area is on your right in front of an old quarry.

Pharaoh Mountain

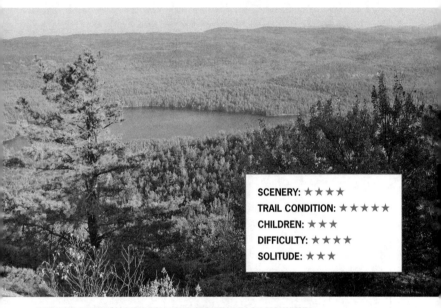

SCENERY: ★ ★ ★ ★
TRAIL CONDITION: ★ ★ ★ ★ ★
CHILDREN: ★ ★ ★
DIFFICULTY: ★ ★ ★ ★
SOLITUDE: ★ ★ ★

LOOKING DOWN ON PHARAOH LAKE FROM PHARAOH MOUNTAIN

GPS COORDINATES: Crane Pond Road parking area: N43° 51.548'   W73° 41.312'

DISTANCE & CONFIGURATION: 9.2-mile out-and-back

HIKING TIME: 6–7 hours

HIGHLIGHTS: Spectacular views, scenic marsh

ELEVATION: 1,060' at trailhead, 2,556' at highest point

ACCESS: Open 24/7; no fees or permits required

MAPS: National Geographic *Adirondack Park, Lake George/Great Sacandaga* (#743)

FACILITIES: None

WHEELCHAIR ACCESS: No

COMMENTS: Accessibility along the rough and partially flooded Crane Pond Road has deteriorated to the point where even high-clearance, four-wheel-drive vehicles frequently get stuck. Plus, driving on the road is illegal. As such, trail directions and mileage have been updated.

CONTACTS: Eastern Adirondack trail information: www.dec.ny.gov/outdoor/9199.html; emergency contact: 518-891-0235

Pharaoh Mountain

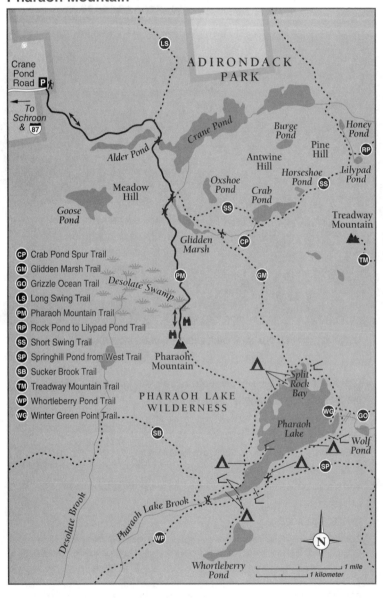

CP Crab Pond Spur Trail
GM Glidden Marsh Trail
GO Grizzle Ocean Trail
LS Long Swing Trail
PM Pharaoh Mountain Trail
RP Rock Pond to Lilypad Pond Trail
SS Short Swing Trail
SP Springhill Pond from West Trail
SB Sucker Brook Trail
TM Treadway Mountain Trail
WP Whortleberry Pond Trail
WG Winter Green Point Trail

Overview

An excellent peak in the eastern section of the Adirondacks, Pharaoh Mountain is an exceptional destination in itself or as a side trip in the heart of the Pharaoh Lake Wilderness. Atop the mountain are great views of the eastern Adirondacks and, on a clear day, the High Peaks to the north as well as the Green Mountains in Vermont. A longer loop is available for hikers who descend to Pharaoh Lake and return via the Glidden Marsh Trail (11.8-mile loop).

Route Details

Crane Pond Road is officially closed at the end of the pavement, where a small parking area has been established. However, in the past locals and others accessing Crane Pond and Pharaoh Lake Wilderness routinely used the unmaintained road. The road was barricaded in the 1980s, but local residents removed the barricade the following spring. When Earth First! tried to erect a new barrier, a conflict arose that involved a pugilistic encounter between a local politician and an Earth First! representative. The whole incident was caught on camera and eventually made it to the national news. At present, there are no barriers, and the road is left open and used by hikers, anglers,

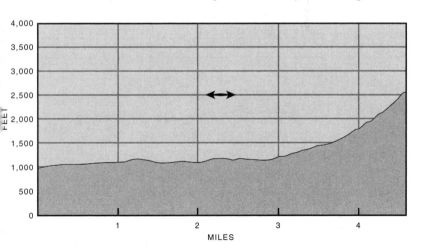

boaters, and campers alike. Be aware that the road is not maintained and is very rough. Even high-clearance, four-wheel-drive vehicles get stuck along the remaining 1.9 miles to the Crane Pond parking area, so I do not recommend planning on driving farther along the road.

Continue south along the rough road as it winds 1.5 miles through a dense forest to where the road descends to a flooded section, which varies in depth and length, depending on recent rain and the season. If you drove farther along the closed road, do not count on being able to drive farther. If you can't cross, there is a bypass trail north of the flooded section. Past the flooded section, the road continues to wind through the forest, passing the Long Swing Trail at 1.7 miles and eventually reaching the first of two grassy parking areas. If you thought one would have to be crazy to ford the flooded section, you will be surprised to find several vehicles that made the crossing.

Proceed east to the boat launch and second parking area, and then head south past a downed pine tree and a trail sign on your right, 1.9 miles. A wide bridge crosses the outlet of Crane Pond, which is on your left, as it flows into Alder Pond on your right. The trail, marked by red disks, uses primarily old access roads, so it is broad and free of obstructions. Additionally, there are very few muddy areas, so this trail is one of the few in the Adirondacks that are in exceptional condition. The wide trail climbs gently as it winds through a mostly hemlock forest a little less than 0.3 mile to the trail register. It continues over level terrain another 0.5 mile under the canopy of towering hemlocks and eastern white pines to a fork in the trail. This intersection, 0.7 mile from Crane Pond, 2.6 miles overall, is situated on the northern tip of Glidden Marsh. Looming straight ahead over the marsh's placid water is Pharaoh Mountain. To the right is the direct approach to the summit, as well as a route to Pharaoh Lake, while on the left is another route to Pharaoh Lake via Glidden Marsh. If you desire a longer trip, descend from the summit to Pharaoh Lake, skirt the lakeshore on the northern trail (not shown on most maps), and then head back along Glidden Marsh Trail for a circuit of 11.1 miles.

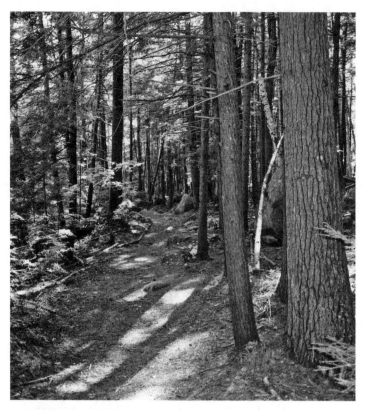

TRAIL TO PHARAOH MOUNTAIN

For a description of the return leg along Glidden Marsh, see the Pharaoh Lake overnight section on page 197.

Bear right at the fork in the trail, and proceed along the western shore of Glidden Marsh. You will cross a couple of log bridges as you navigate the next 0.3 mile over level terrain. At 2.9 miles, the climb to the summit begins. As you ascend, the forest transitions from the towering evergreens to a mostly hardwood forest. The mixture features oak and cherry trees at first, and then gives way to predominantly maple and beech. At 3.6 miles, you reach a fork with an overgrown abandoned road on the left, but the trail continues on your right. The easy hiking along old roads gives way to rougher hiking as you pick your way along exposed bedrock and through the rocks and cobbles that dominate the trail. Approximately 3.9 miles in, the canopy height begins to diminish and the forest transitions back to evergreens, though the composition is now stunted firs dotted with birches.

At 4.2 miles, you will have to rock-hop across a stream, and the climbing becomes much steeper. Over the next 0.5 mile, the trees become stunted, and the trail, flanked by alpine mosses, crosses over exposed portions of bedrock. As you approach the summit, several exposed ledges are either on the trail or mere feet to your right, with amazing views to the north and west. I suggest taking some time to admire the views to the north, as the panorama at the summit is mostly to the west and south. At the summit, the trail passes through a shallow cleft that bisects what are essentially the two summits of Pharaoh Mountain. The northern knob is to your left and has exceptional views to the west, especially of Schroon Lake. Footpaths meander about the northern knob, where a couple of informal campsites are interspersed among the windswept firs. Follow the main path a very short distance south to find the footpath that leads to the southern knob. The exposed portions of bedrock on this knob offer incredible views of Pharaoh Lake.

Note: The Pharaoh Lake overnight trail begins at the end of this trail.

Directions

From I-87, take Exit 28, and head east on NY 74. Immediately turn right onto US 9 in Schroon Lake. In 0.6 mile turn left onto Alder Meadow Road. Follow Alder Meadow Road 2.1 miles, and bear left onto Crane Pond Road. The parking lot is on the left where the pavement ends and Crane Pond Road turns into an unmaintained road at 1.4 miles.

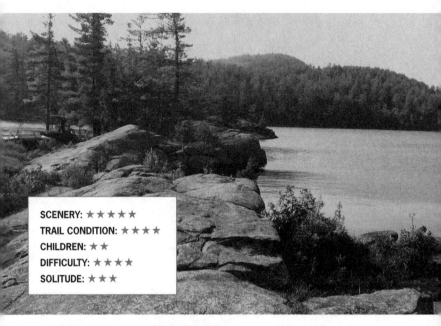

SCENERY: ★ ★ ★ ★ ★
TRAIL CONDITION: ★ ★ ★ ★
CHILDREN: ★ ★
DIFFICULTY: ★ ★ ★ ★
SOLITUDE: ★ ★ ★

WINTER GREEN POINT ON PHARAOH LAKE

GPS COORDINATES: Crane Pond Road parking area: N43° 51.548'   W73° 41.312'

DISTANCE & CONFIGURATION: 17.3-mile loop

HIKING TIME: Overnight

HIGHLIGHTS: Exceptional lakeside camping, waterfall

ELEVATION: 2,500' at trailhead (at the end of Pharaoh Mountain Trail), 992' at lowest point

ACCESS: Open 24/7; no fees or permits required

MAPS: National Geographic *Adirondack Park, Lake George/Great Sacandaga* (#743)

FACILITIES: None

WHEELCHAIR ACCESS: No

COMMENTS: The trail description presumes access via the Pharaoh Mountain Trail. Bypassing the summit via the Glidden Marsh Trail cuts 1.5 miles and 1,000 feet of elevation change from the hike.

CONTACTS: Eastern Adirondack trail information: www.dec.ny.gov/outdoor/9199.html; emergency contact: 518-891-0235

Pharaoh Lake

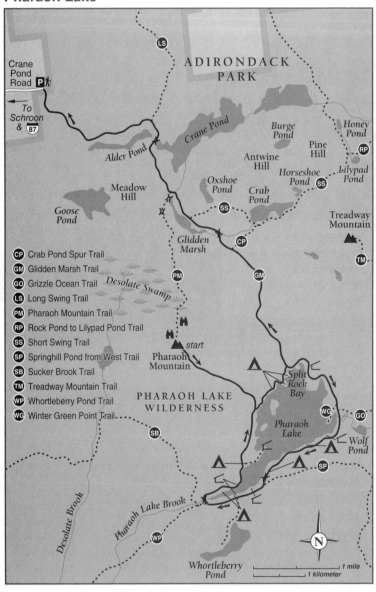

ADIRONDACK PARK

Crane Pond Road

To Schroon & 87

PHARAOH LAKE WILDERNESS

CP Crab Pond Spur Trail
GM Glidden Marsh Trail
GO Grizzle Ocean Trail
LS Long Swing Trail
PM Pharaoh Mountain Trail
RP Rock Pond to Lilypad Pond Trail
SS Short Swing Trail
SP Springhill Pond from West Trail
SB Sucker Brook Trail
TM Treadway Mountain Trail
WP Whortleberry Pond Trail
WG Winter Green Point Trail

Crane Pond
Alder Pond
Meadow Hill
Goose Pond
Glidden Marsh
Desolate Swamp
Pharaoh Mountain
start
Burge Pond
Antwine Hill
Oxshoe Pond
Crab Pond
Pine Hill
Horseshoe Pond
Honey Pond
Lilypad Pond
Treadway Mountain
Split Rock Bay
Pharaoh Lake
Wolf Pond
Desolate Brook
Pharaoh Lake Brook
Whortleberry Pond

1 mile
1 kilometer

Overview

The lean-tos and designated campsites along the shores of Pharaoh Lake are some of the best in the Adirondacks. The sheer number of sites in this virtual wilderness campground means that you will likely find a spot even on busy holiday weekends. If you crave solitude, choose an off-peak weekend or shy away from the lean-tos and pick a remote tent site. The designated sites and lean-tos are nearly all next to the shore with scenic views, and it's clear why they are popular.

Route Details

Numerous trails lead to Pharaoh Lake, but the description provided here is from the end of Pharaoh Mountain Trail, described on page 191. Bear in mind that parking for the Pharaoh Mountain Trailhead along the unmaintained portion of Crane Pond Road is no longer recommended or feasible. See the Pharaoh Mountain Trail description for details.

From the end of Pharaoh Mountain Trail, descend the southern slope following the red trail markers, 4.6 miles from the end of the paved portion of Crane Pond Road. Shortly after leaving the summit, you must climb down a vertical portion of exposed ledge that

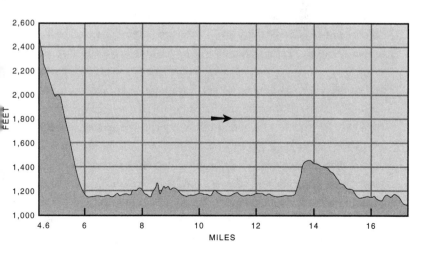

is several feet high and requires the use of both hands. Footholds are available in a small cleft next to the adjoining sheer rock face on your right. The descent is steeper than the climb to the summit, and the forest quickly transforms from alpine evergreens and birches to dense maples and beeches. At 6.2 miles, a sheer cliff looms to your right and indicates that you are nearing the lakeshore. Soon after, you traverse a wet section across planks laid lengthwise. By now, you can catch masked glimpses of the lake through the thick beech saplings.

At 6.4 miles, you reach the intersection with the north lakeside trail. From here, you can circle the lake in either direction. Counterclockwise, to your right, is the fastest and most direct approach to the majority of the lean-tos. On the other hand, heading clockwise brings you to some of the best campsites, as well as Split Rock Bay and the final return route via Glidden Marsh; this northern section of the trail is not shown on most maps of the area. The description and mileage here are given for the clockwise direction.

Turn left and follow the west-shore trail, marked with blue disks, toward Split Rock Bay. This portion of the trail is roughly 0.7 mile long and follows the shoreline very closely. It also features three great designated camping areas. The first of these is just off the trail at 6.6 miles. A fire pit has been placed along an exposed portion of ledge within feet of the lake, and a long, rocky peninsula makes a superb spot to admire the view. A little less than 0.3 mile ahead, you will pass a yellow Department of Environmental Conservation designated camping disk with an arrow. These arrow disks indicate that a designated site is nearby. Usually these sites are farther off the trail and can be easily located by following the arrows. On occasion, disks will be missing or the indicated direction of the arrow may lead you astray, so use the disks as a means to zero in on the spot rather than as absolute markers. In this case, wander out along the southern edge of the peninsula, just below an elevated ridge, and you will find the picturesque site. Surrounded by tall pines and small blueberry bushes, it sits high on the elevated peninsula and offers commanding views of the lake.

Back along the loop, the trail dips down and follows a cattail-filled bay briefly before reaching another designated camping disk at 6.9 miles. To reach this site, head east onto another small peninsula, where you will find a site very similar to the last one near the peninsula's tip. The intersection with Glidden Marsh Trail back to Crane Pond is at 7 miles.

Shortly after the intersection, the trail, now marked in yellow, winds along another bay with large boulders sticking up in the middle. This is Split Rock Bay, and while the rocks do look split from this shore, their appearance from the opposite shore is more dramatic. From that shore, the split rocks appear to be a pair of obelisks with an eerie and unnatural quality. On your way to the opposite shore, you will pass an abandoned fiberglass boat, which, had you come from the other direction, would not seem unusual. At 7.6 miles, you reach Lean-To 4 (also known as Split Rock Bay Lean-To), which is within a couple dozen feet of the shore and has an open view south out onto the lake.

It's likely that you will see a boat pulled up on the shore nearby, and the mystery of the abandoned boat will start to resolve itself. In fact, all the lean-tos around the lake have some sort of boat, usually a canoe or small rowboat, located nearby. Improvised paddles are typically found nearby as well, but they are, in some cases, little more than flat logs. If you have the foresight to pack an ultralight paddle, you could easily become the most popular guest at the lake.

The trail swings northeast at the lean-to and heads into a thick hemlock forest. This area is heavily shaded and has few saplings, so the views into the surrounding forest are expansive. Dotted with mossy, wet areas, this brief foray into a hemlock swamp is a pleasant change of pace from the standard hardwoods, but the trail delves back into mixed hardwoods after 0.4 mile. At 8.3 miles, you reach another intersection. To your right is a side trip to Winter Green Point, marked with red disks, while straight ahead is the continuation of the lakeside trail. The less than 0.3-mile side trip to the rocky point is definitely worthwhile and provides views of the lake as well as Pharaoh Mountain.

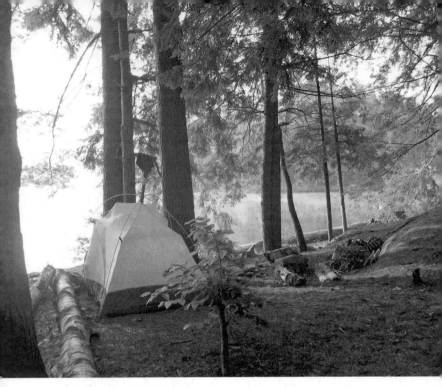

CAMPSITE ON PHARAOH LAKE

Back on the trail, you quickly reach another fork; to the left are Grizzle Ocean and Putnam Pond Campground, 5.8 miles away, while the lakeside trail continues straight ahead. Roughly 0.3 mile ahead, you reach a wide stream crossing where the log cribbing is all that remains of an old bridge. You can easily rock-hop across, but you might want to bushwhack a short distance upstream to where a tiny waterfall splashes into a deep, boulder-dammed pool. The trail winds up and down a few hillocks through a mixed pine forest before reaching another intersection at 8.6 miles. Lean-To 3 is off to your right, while the east-shore trail continues ahead. The lean-to sits on an elevated cliff along the lake and offers outstanding views. Before finally dropping to the lakeshore, the ledge has several wide step-downs, all of which make excellent spots to dally.

The trail continues southwest among the mixed pines for a while, and you reach another designated campsite at 9 miles. The site is just off the trail but is quite close to the lake and is a good spot for anyone wishing to avoid the crowds that congregate at lean-tos. From this point on, many portions of the east-shore trail hug the shoreline, and views of Pharaoh Mountain are superb. Highbush blueberries crowd the trail along the exposed portions of lichen-covered ledge that form the shoreline and much of the trail. At 9.3 miles, you cross a plank bridge to a small peninsula and pass an informal campsite that sees regular use. A quarter mile later you pass a designated campsite with exceptional views of Pharaoh Mountain across the lake.

You reach another major intersection at 9.9 miles. To the left and marked in red are Springhill Pond, 4.5 miles, and New Hague Road, 8.3 miles, while the east-shore trail continues straight ahead, still marked in yellow. Shortly ahead, you reach Lean-To 2. This is the largest of the lean-tos—double the capacity of the others—with a pleasant grassy field sloping down to the lake in front of it. The view is less desirable than in other locations but seems very popular nonetheless. The trail toward the outlet and Lean-To 1 is an old road that passes through a tall hemlock-and-pine forest. The wide road is free of obstructions and allows deep views into the surrounding forest. As you come down a slight hill, you see the side of Lean-To 1. Close to the shore, it has beautiful views of the north shore and, like the rest of the lean-tos, has a watercraft stowed nearby.

The wide road continues south to the outlet of the lake, but you have to pass through a long mire before the canopy opens up at the grassy southern tip of the lake, 10.7 miles. The trail, now marked with red disks, heads north along the lakeshore, and you quickly reach another yellow camping disk with an arrow indicating a site nearby. The site lies atop the small knoll to your right. Though it's high above the water, views of the lake are shielded by a rise in the hill and the saplings that line the hill. Nonetheless, it is a fine site and ideal for those seeking privacy and a sheltered setting. A little more than 0.3 mile from the outlet, you reach a fork in the trail; veer left to follow the trail, or head right following yellow disks to Lean-To 6. Though it is situated more than 100 yards from the lakeshore, it has excellent views, and the deep evergreen forest that shades the site makes it feel uniquely isolated.

The trail continues north, winding through hemlock groves along the lakeshore and up into deciduous hilltops. At 11.4 miles, you pass another designated site, which is situated on the forest side of the trail. This is probably the least desirable of the sites but would make a good stopping point if the lean-tos are full and night is coming on. At 11.6 miles, you reach yet another fork in the trail. To your left is the main trail, while straight ahead is Lean-To 5 (also known as Watch Rocks Lean-To). The lean-to trail is marked in yellow and closely follows the shoreline. Located near the tip of the peninsula, it has views in all directions, the most exceptional being at the point itself.

The main trail, rougher here than in other sections, climbs slightly and weaves its way mostly through a thick hardwood forest. The lake is no longer visible, and there is very little of note until you return to the intersection with Pharaoh Mountain Trail, 12.4 miles. Continue until you reach the intersection with Glidden Marsh Trail, 13 miles. Emblazoned with yellow disks, Glidden Marsh Trail climbs away from the lake immediately. The rocky climb is through mostly deciduous forest, and there are noticeably more ash trees along the slope than elsewhere along the hike. After roughly 0.3 mile, the trail levels off as you begin to pass a broad wetland on your right. The wetland, the result of beaver activity, becomes quite broad, and the trail often passes through its muddy edges for the next mile. The trail leaves the marshy section and reenters the forest as you begin a 0.3-mile descent to another fork in the trail. Straight ahead and marked in yellow is Crane Pond, while off to the right is Crab Pond Spur Trail that passes Crab and Horseshoe Ponds.

Shortly after this intersection at 14.6 miles, a log bridge spans a feeder stream of Glidden Marsh, and you reach the eastern shore of the marsh soon after. The trail closely follows the broad, grassy marshland, where you can see several beaver lodges in the center of the deeper water. At 15.2 miles, you come to the intersection with Short Swing Trail, which passes Oxshoe Pond, on your right. The main

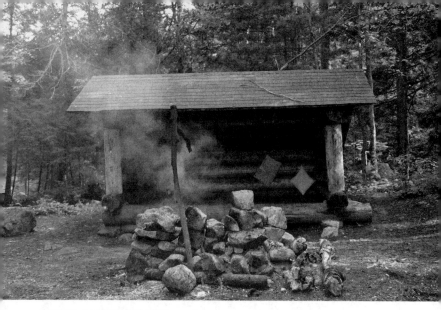

LEAN-TO 4 AT PHARAOH LAKE

trail, Glidden Marsh Trail, and Short Swing Trail are marked with blue disks. You lose sight of Glidden Marsh as you pass on the eastern side of a small hill that flanks the marsh. Another marsh down to your right is a dammed stream that feeds Crane Pond before the trail turns west. The trail crosses a log bridge and then climbs a rocky hill before descending to the intersection with Pharaoh Mountain Trail. Heading north on the old, abandoned road, the mileage is as follows: less than 0.5 mile to the trail register, 0.7 mile to the Crane Pond parking area, and 2.6 miles to the designated parking area. This section of the trail is marked with red disks and is easy to follow, but for a more thorough description, read the Pharaoh Mountain Trail section.

Directions

From I-87, take Exit 28, and head east on NY 74. Immediately turn right onto US 9 in Schroon Lake. In 0.6 mile turn left onto Alder Meadow Road. Follow Alder Meadow Road 2.1 miles, and bear left onto Crane Pond Road. The parking lot is on the left where the pavement ends and Crane Pond Road turns into an unmaintained road at 1.4 miles.

Northern (Hikes 30–36)

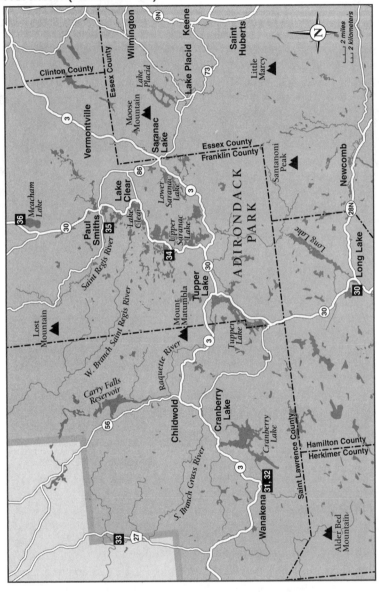

Northern

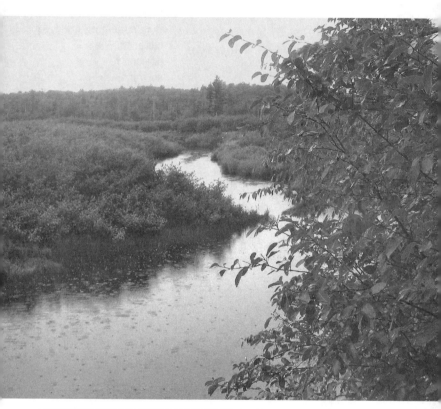

OSWEGATCHIE RIVER SEEN FROM HIGH ROCK *(Trail 32, High Falls, page 218)*

Owls Head Mountain

SCENERY: ★ ★ ★ ★ ★
TRAIL CONDITION: ★ ★ ★ ★
CHILDREN: ★ ★ ★ ★
DIFFICULTY: ★ ★ ★
SOLITUDE: ★ ★ ★ ★

VISTA FROM ATOP OWLS HEAD FIRE TOWER

GPS COORDINATES: N43° 57.812'   W74° 27.173'

DISTANCE & CONFIGURATION: 6.3-mile out-and-back

HIKING TIME: 3–4 hours

HIGHLIGHTS: Panoramic views, fire tower, historic site

ELEVATION: 1,665' at trailhead, 2,762' at highest point

ACCESS: Open 24/7; no fees or permits required

MAPS: National Geographic *Adirondack Park, Old Forge/Oswegatchie* (#745)

FACILITIES: None

WHEELCHAIR ACCESS: No

CONTACTS: Emergency contact: 518-891-0235

Overview

On the boundary of the west-central and northern sections of the Adirondacks is scenic Owls Head. By climbing the accessible fire tower on the summit, you have a 360-degree view of the surrounding hills and lakes. The remains of an old observer cabin add historical interest.

Route Details

The trailhead and register are located on the left side of the small parking pullout. The parking area is located on a curve along Endion Lane and may accommodate a dozen cars if visitors park thoughtfully. The trail, marked with red disks, immediately begins to ascend amid a dense maple-and-beech hardwood forest. After 0.3 mile the trail levels off and follows mostly rolling terrain another 1.3 miles. At 1 mile from the trailhead, you reach an intersection with another trail. To your left is the trail to Owls Head summit, 2.1 miles away, while to your right is a trail to NY 30, 3.5 miles, and Lake Eaton Campground, 3.8 miles. Shortly after the first intersection, you pass an abandoned foot trail on your right, followed by an old road that joins the main trail from behind. The old road has orange placards with white diamonds. A few of these placards, as well as snowmobile disks, are interspersed with the red Department of Environmental Conservation trail markers along the main trail. Aside from the previously mentioned intersections, the trail runs in a relatively straight southwest direction to the summit and is easy to follow.

At 2 miles, the trail swings south and begins to ascend gradually and then more steeply at 2.3 miles. A seasonal stream flows on your left as you climb through sections of heavy erosion. You reach a crest in the trail at 2.7 miles. You have not yet reached the summit but are passing between two points along the mountain that resemble the horns of an owl. The trail dips down, less than 100 feet of elevation, into a small valley before climbing steeply to the summit. Before you make the final ascent, you pass by the former site of the cabin used by the fire tower's observer.

Owls Head Mountain

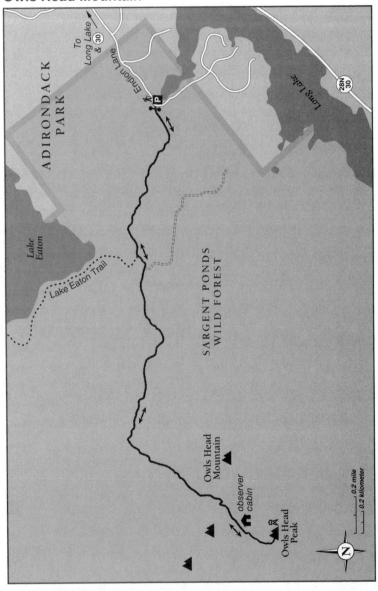

Around the turn of the 20th century, forest fires swept the Adirondack region, and nearly 1 million acres of forest burned throughout the preserve. In response to this destruction, the state erected fire towers atop many peaks throughout the Adirondacks. The tasks of state-employed observers included locating and triangulating fires. On the side, they also provided innumerable hikers with information and conservation education. A wooden fire tower was erected on the peak of Owls Head around 1911. It was replaced by a steel tower in 1919 and closed in 1979. After restoration work was complete, it was reopened in 2004, and efforts are currently under way to continue maintenance of the tower.

The final climb to the summit passes over exposed portions of ledge and includes multiple small switchbacks. You will need to use both hands in several sections. The trail suddenly ends as you come through a thick stand of firs near the base of the steel fire tower. Multiple grassy patches threaded through the exposed portions of the summit (elevation: 2,812') make excellent picnic areas. A large slab of exposed rock juts out to the southwest, providing an outstanding lookout. For a 360-degree view of the area, you should climb the fire tower. The fence-enclosed stairs lead to a wooden platform covered by a steel cap typical of the fire towers still in use in the Adirondacks.

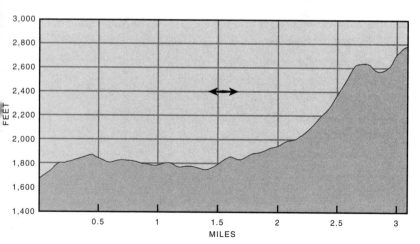

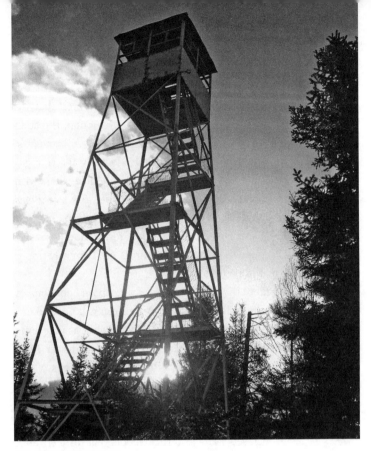

OWLS HEAD FIRE TOWER

On your way up, you may have seen old utility poles alongside the trail. If not, they are more noticeable on your way back down. The two opposing "branches" on these poles also resemble owls' horns, making the name of this trail doubly apt.

Directions

From the north intersection of NY 30 and NY 28N in Long Lake, head northwest on NY 30. In 1.3 miles turn left onto Endion Lane. Follow Endion Lane 1.6 miles, and look for the gravel pullout on the right.

Cat Mountain

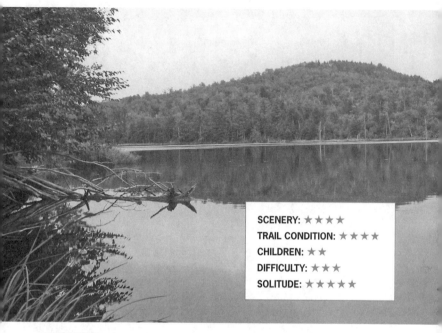

SCENERY: ★ ★ ★ ★
TRAIL CONDITION: ★ ★ ★ ★
CHILDREN: ★ ★
DIFFICULTY: ★ ★ ★
SOLITUDE: ★ ★ ★ ★ ★

GLASBY POND

GPS COORDINATES: N44° 07.989' W74° 54.915'

DISTANCE & CONFIGURATION: 9.7-mile out-and-back (from Wanakena) or 4.8-mile out-and-back (if boating to Janacks Landing)

HIKING TIME: 5–6 hours

HIGHLIGHTS: Scenic pond, beautiful vistas

ELEVATION: 1,502' at trailhead, 2,260' at highest point

ACCESS: Open 24/7; no fees or permits required

MAPS: Five Ponds Wilderness map: tinyurl.com/5pondsmap; National Geographic *Adirondack Park, Old Forge/Oswegatchie* (#745)

FACILITIES: None

WHEELCHAIR ACCESS: No

CONTACTS: Five Ponds Wilderness: www.dec.ny.gov/lands/34719.html; emergency contact: 518-891-0235

Cat Mountain

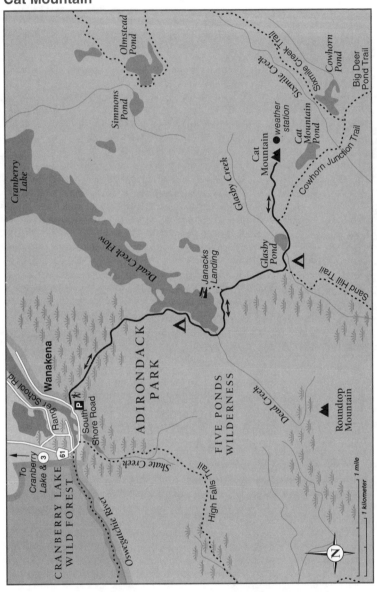

Overview

Cat Mountain is a beautiful little peak that offers excellent views. Combined with the High Falls overnighter, it makes a nice side trip or an extended day trip on its own. To add a bit more adventure to the hike, you can boat in from Cranberry Lake to Janacks Landing and bypass roughly 5 miles of the round-trip hike.

Route Details

Hike in from the western terminus of the High Falls Loop in Wanakena or boat to Janacks Landing in the Dead Creek Flow arm of Cranberry Lake. The trail described here will be from Wanakena with a side note about boat access; boaters can pick up the trail and follow the description from the Janacks Landing intersection.

The trail and register are elevated a few feet above the spacious parking area on the southern edge. The trail begins heading east but quickly swings south along an abandoned logging road. The wide and flat roadbed, over relatively level terrain, allows for easy hiking for the first 2 miles. You will make quick time, except where flooding due to beaver activity inundates the trail. You will encounter several mires, as well as sections of knee-deep water. The nearly

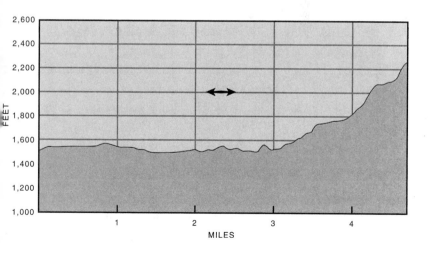

black, murky waters are deceptive: most of the time the water is less than 1 inch deep when it flows over the berms and beaver dams, but occasional breaks in dams and the soft mud underfoot can lead to drops of 1 foot or more, with little evidence provided by the placid waters. Hiking sticks act as probes in questionable spots and, as is the case at most trailheads, previous hikers typically leave decent sticks at the trail register.

The road, emblazoned with red disks, gently descends most of the way, and at approximately 1.5 miles, the waters of Dead Creek Flow become visible. The road closely follows the shoreline 0.4 mile, at which point you come across a large campsite. Boaters often use this and the other 46 designated primitive sites along the lakeshore. At this point, the road ends, and the trail becomes a typical Adirondack trail. It crosses Dead Creek at 2.3 miles and then swings around the bay of Dead Creek Flow and heads east 0.5 mile.

After the short easterly jog along the trail, you intersect the Janacks Landing Trail. The trail is now heading nearly due south and gradually climbs to Sand Hill Junction. The climb is steady and crisscrosses a small stream in several places before reaching a junction at 3.6 miles. Straight ahead is the easterly leg of the High Falls Loop, while the Cat Mountain summit and Glasby Pond are to your left along the Cowhorn Junction Trail.

The trail, marked with yellow disks, climbs steadily along Glasby Creek past a few small cascades, and the rush of water on your right is a pleasant addition to the trail. After passing through a small, bramble-filled meadow, you come out on the western shores of Glasby Pond at 3.8 miles. The steep cliffs of Cat Mountain provide a striking view across the pristine waters. You will pass through a large campsite before weaving your way up and over a tiny hillock, after which the pondside trail becomes a continuous mire. The terrain grows steadily steeper as you head away from the pond, and you soon reach the final fork in the trail. The Cowhorn Junction Trail continues off to your right toward Cowhorn and Cat Mountain Ponds, marked by yellow disks; to reach the Cat Mountain summit, veer left and follow the red trail markers.

The next 0.6 mile to the summit is the steepest section, and the trail is a mix of short scrambles over bedrock and boulder-strewn steps. The hardwoods at the base of the mountain give way to windswept evergreens as you weave your way through small switchbacks. Paths on the left reach a few rocky outlooks. These offer nice views, but the best are available at the summit. The trail finally winds its way out onto the southern clifftops. You'll find a solar-powered weather station and the remnants of an old fire tower here at the trail end. Enjoy beautiful views on this portion of the cliffs, or search for better ones by dipping into the coppice of evergreens behind you and making your way along paths to the next section of the clifftop. The drop-off to the south is quite sheer, allowing spectacular views down to Cat Mountain Pond as well as Roundtop and Threemile Mountains along the horizon.

A note about boat access: A public boat launch is located just off NY 3, on Columbian Road near Cranberry Lake's dam in the village of Cranberry Lake. The hard-surface launch can accommodate trailer launches and, according to the Department of Environmental Conservation, can fit 55 vehicles. Navigating from the launch site to Janacks Landing should not be too difficult if you follow the western shore into Dead Creek Flow Bay.

Directions

From the intersection of NY 3 and Youngs Road in Star Lake, head 6.1 miles east on NY 3, and then follow the directions below. From the intersection of NY 3 and Lone Pine Road in Cranberry Lake, head 8.3 miles west on NY 3, and follow the directions below.

Turn southeast onto County Road 61/Main Street. Bear right at 0.8 mile onto Main Street, which becomes South Shore Road; continue 0.5 mile and cross the steel bridge over the Oswegatchie River. After the bridge, go another 0.5 mile, and the parking area and trailhead are on the right.

32 High Falls

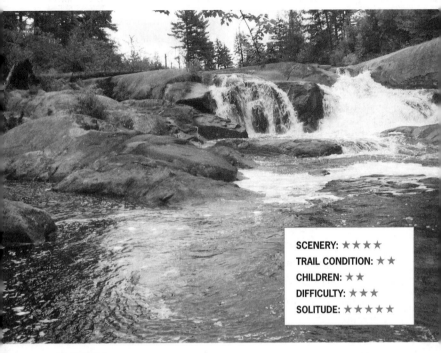

SCENERY: ★ ★ ★ ★
TRAIL CONDITION: ★ ★
CHILDREN: ★ ★
DIFFICULTY: ★ ★ ★
SOLITUDE: ★ ★ ★ ★ ★

HIGH FALLS

GPS COORDINATES: N44° 07.911'   W74° 55.383'

DISTANCE & CONFIGURATION: 16.2-mile loop

HIKING TIME: Overnight

HIGHLIGHTS: Isolated waterfall, numerous beaver dams, wetlands and ponds, winding-flat river, lakeside hiking, berry picking

ELEVATION: 1,490' at trailhead, 1,660' at highest point

ACCESS: Open 24/7; no fees or permits required

MAPS: Five Ponds Wilderness map: tinyurl.com/5pondsmap; National Geographic *Adirondack Park, Old Forge/Oswegatchie* (#745)

FACILITIES: None

WHEELCHAIR ACCESS: No

CONTACTS: Five Ponds Wilderness: www.dec.ny.gov/lands/34719.html; emergency contact: 518-891-0235

Overview

With a wide variety of habitats and mostly easy trekking, this is a great introductory backpacking trip. Beaver activity is practically every-where, with several dam tops forming part of the trail, so don't expect to keep your feet dry for long. In midsummer, the abundance of blue-berries practically turns foraging into hike-by food service.

Route Details

Parking is available on either end of the loop, with roughly 0.5 mile of road in between. You will have to make the roadside trek either before or after your wilderness experience. With merely 0.5 mile and limited parking in each area, the use of two cars seems extravagant. My recommendation is to stow your pack at the trailhead on which you wish to start, park at the other trailhead, and walk back to your desired start. You can hike the trail in either direction: heading coun-terclockwise, High Falls is 9.0 miles; heading clockwise, it is 6.5 miles. You can add a side trip to Cat Mountain (described on page 213) to the clockwise approach or on the return, making the mileage on the eastern leg the same. I recommend camping at High Falls, but if time or weather forces you to camp early, designated riverside campsites (briefly described below) are located along the western leg, while camp-ing along the eastern leg will require short bushwhacks to adhere to Department of Environmental Conservation (DEC) wilderness camp-ing regulations. Trail directions below are heading counterclockwise.

From the western parking area, walk around the tennis court down the private road to a vehicle-barrier gate just past a residence on your right. The trail register is a little beyond the barrier and has a map of the area, including 46 designated campsites along the Oswegatchie River. Most of these sites are either across the river or require bushwhacking, so these are mainly used by canoeists and kayakers. The first mile of the trail is along a grass-covered gravel road, which provides access for municipal water. With the trail free of any obstructions, you will have the opportunity to look out for

High Falls

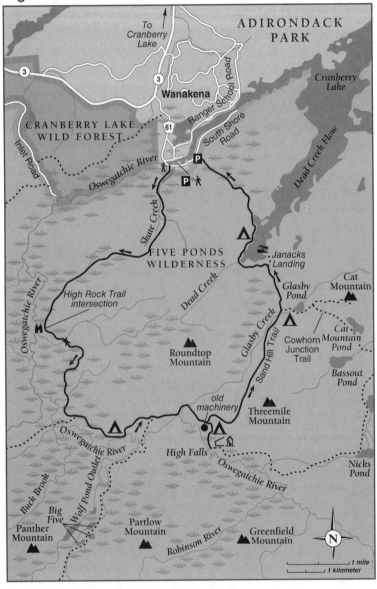

wildlife in the dammed section of Skate Creek on your left. A little more than 0.5 mile in, you will cross Skate Creek, and its wetland will sprawl off to your right. These broad, marshy areas are very common in the northern section of the Adirondacks and are often seen from the road but are not frequently traversable on foot.

Approximately 1 mile in, the trail crosses a stream that feeds into Skate Creek and begins to climb as you plunge into a mixed hardwood forest. It would be hard to get lost along this wide-open road, but red DEC markers assure you that you are headed in the right direction. At 1.8 miles, you will come to a clearing where an overgrown road climbs to your left. In the past, numerous roads and paths headed more directly to the High Falls area, but the microburst windstorm of 1995 created so much blowdown that these trails have been abandoned. Beyond the clearing, ferns and other deciduous plants encroach on the trail, but its past use as a road is unmistakable, as it is broad, flat, and free of typical obstructions and is elevated above the surrounding terrain. The western half of the trail consists almost entirely of abandoned roads, which makes its 9.0 miles nearly equivalent in effort to the 6.5-mile hike along the eastern leg.

At 2.3 miles, the canopy opens, and another creek with a broad wetland sprawls out on your right. Despite being flanked by

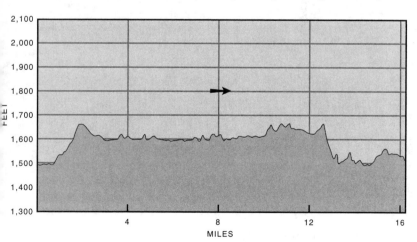

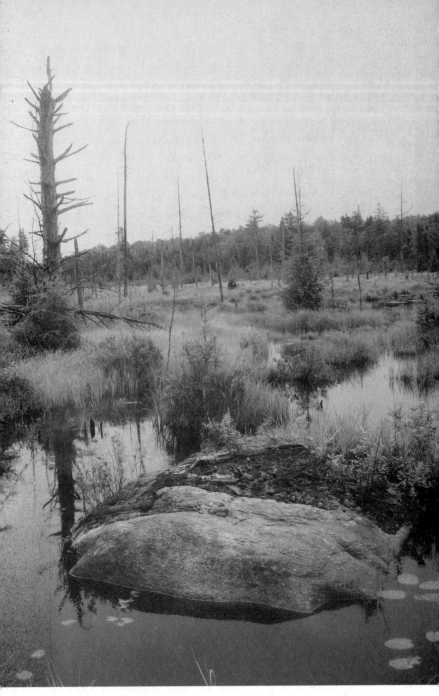

ONE OF THE MANY AREAS THAT HAVE FLOODED DUE TO BEAVER ACTIVITY short evergreens, the trail is open to the sky. At this point, you have reached the plateau that the western leg traverses, and the rest of the way gently rolls along at this elevation. During the summer, the trailside will be thick with highbush blueberries.

At 3.8 miles, you reenter the hardwood forest and come to a fork in the trail. High Rock, which overlooks the Oswegatchie River, is 0.1 mile to your right. The boulder that provides an outlook across the meandering river is actually not very high. However, the plain through which the river cuts its veritable maze is so broad that you can see quite far. A popular campsite is also located here, so do not be surprised to see your first group of boaters. Though the Oswegatchie flows north to the west of the trail, this side trip will be your only opportunity to see it for several miles.

Heading south, you walk over a stone-and-concrete bridge that spans a stream at 4.3 miles. At 5.3 miles, you encounter the first of many beaver dams that have created wide marshlands both up- and downstream. To cross this and future dammed sections, you will walk along the tops of the dams. Picking your way atop the dams is not difficult, but wet feet are inevitable. Aside from the wet areas created by the beaver dams, the trail is relatively level and easygoing along these old logging roads. Less than 1 mile ahead, mile 6.1, you traverse another dammed section, and then shortly after reenter the forest.

In 0.5 mile the trail meets the Oswegatchie, as well as the first of three easily accessible designated campsites along the river. The first site, with no number, is directly on the trail, while a short way ahead a path leads to site 28, which is masked by a stand of thick saplings. This site also has the advantage of sitting just above a small flume that adds interest to the mostly flat river.

Shortly after this brief encounter with the river, you head back into wetland territory along another stream and then back into the forest, where you reach a fork in the trail, 7.5 miles. Trail signs indicate that High Falls is 1.5 miles ahead, while the fork to the right takes you deep into the Five Ponds Wilderness. Shortly ahead, you enter an area where Glasby Creek and the Oswegatchie River meet.

This confluence creates a broad wetland and meadow setting with beaver activity throughout. Yellow disks indicate a couple of designated campsites in the area, but their locations escaped me. Many of the designated campsites either were affected by the 1995 microburst storm or see little use because most people are headed to the High Falls lean-tos or campsites. After crossing a log-and-plank bridge, the trail climbs through a short section of stunted pines that gradually gives way to mixed hardwoods.

At mile 8.6 you reach an intersection; High Falls is 0.5 mile to the right, while it is 6.1 miles back to Wanakena along the eastern leg. Along the trail to High Falls, you will come upon an abandoned and heavily rusted piece of machinery. Its presence adds a quaint reminder that, not too long ago, this area was used by industry, but the wilderness quickly reestablishes itself and wipes out all but the most persistent traces of human activity. After a brief climb, you will hear High Falls and then come to designated campsite 16 and the confluence of several paths, 9.1 miles. The trail directly to the right is the canoe carry that bypasses the falls. A path slightly to your right leads to a boulder at the base of the falls. A path to the left leads to one of the pit toilets in the area. The path straight ahead leads to the start of the canoe carry, the top of the falls, and the lean-to on this side of the river. The falls are only 20 feet tall but are still excellent. The water bifurcates, forming a spray on the left and a rushing torrent on the right. The pool at the base is deep enough to swim in, and while I was there, a heron fishing for brown trout occupied it.

The return trip along the eastern leg is a sharp contrast to the easy hiking along the old logging roads of the western leg. However, it is no different from typical trails in the Adirondacks, except perhaps for the vast amount of beaver activity. Following blue DEC disks, head east from the junction with the western leg; total mileage before starting this leg is 9.6 miles. After picking your way up and over a hillock, where damage from the 1995 microburst storm is still evident, you reach a broad wetland in less than 0.5 mile. A large fallen pine tree forms a bridge over the stream, which should be carefully negotiated,

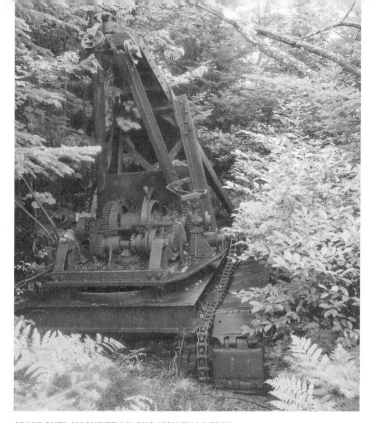

ABANDONED MACHINERY ALONG HIGH FALLS TRAIL

especially when wet. The next 2.2 miles take you along the base of Threemile Mountain through myriad wetlands created by successive beaver dams. The mix of forest and open marshlands created by the beaver dams creates some very interesting scenery complemented by abundant opportunities to pick berries, including blueberries, raspberries, blackcaps, and blackberries, depending on the season.

At 12.2 miles you reach the intersection of the eastern leg, with Cowhorn Junction Trail on the right. This intersection is Sand Hill Junction, where a side trip up to Cat Mountain is highly recommended. Red DEC disks now mark the trail, and you will be heading generally north as the trail begins to descend. You will have to negotiate a few more wet areas before reaching a trail register at the intersection with Janacks Landing Trail. Less than 0.3 mile to the right is a lean-to and boat landing for hikers who wish to boat in and avoid the initial 2.8 miles of the hike along the eastern leg. The nearest boat launch is 7.8 miles away, as the crow flies, in the village of Cranberry Lake; the boat launch is off NY 3 near the dam. Most of the remaining hike is along old logging roads, so hiking in is likely the fastest and most direct approach.

From the intersection, the trail veers west 0.5 mile, where it crosses Dead Creek Flow, which is the largest submerged bay of Cranberry Lake. The distinction may sound peculiar until you realize that this bay was previously the creekbed until Cranberry Lake was dammed in 1867. The hike around the western point of Dead Creek Flow adds yet another scenic element. After coming around the western point, you reach a large designated campground and the beginning of the old logging road, which will take you back to Wanakena. The road climbs with a gentle grade, and you will encounter a few more beaver-flooded areas before reaching the eastern parking area at 16.2 miles.

Directions

From the intersection of NY 3 and Youngs Road in Star Lake, head 6.1 miles east on NY 3, and then follow the directions below. From the intersection of NY 3 and Lone Pine Road in Cranberry Lake, head 8.3 miles west on NY 3, and follow the directions below.

Turn southeast onto County Road 61/Main Street. Bear right at 0.8 mile onto Main Street, which becomes South Shore Road; continue 0.5 mile to cross the steel bridge over the Oswegatchie River. The western trailhead is accessed along a dirt road 0.1 mile past the bridge and on the right. The closest parking area to this trailhead is a little farther along South Shore Road, also on the right just past the tennis court. The eastern trailhead and its parking area are 0.5 mile past the bridge on the right side of the road.

Lampson Falls
and Grass River

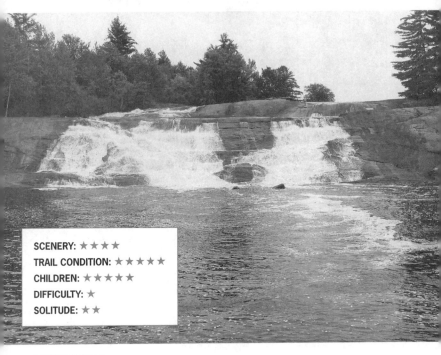

SCENERY: ★ ★ ★ ★
TRAIL CONDITION: ★ ★ ★ ★ ★
CHILDREN: ★ ★ ★ ★ ★
DIFFICULTY: ★
SOLITUDE: ★ ★

LAMPSON FALLS

GPS COORDINATES: N44° 24.302'   W75° 03.680'

DISTANCE & CONFIGURATION: 1.0-mile out-and-back to falls, 3.0-mile out-and-back including riverside trail

HIKING TIME: 1–2 hours

HIGHLIGHTS: Waterfall, riverside walk

ELEVATION: 820' at trailhead, 740' at lowest point

ACCESS: Open 24/7; no fees or permits required

MAPS: National Geographic *Adirondack Park, Saranac/Paul Smiths* (#746)

FACILITIES: None

WHEELCHAIR ACCESS: Yes, on the section of the trail leading to the waterfall lookout

CONTACTS: Northern Adirondack trail information: www.dec.ny.gov/outdoor/9196.html; emergency contact: 518-891-0235

Lampson Falls and Grass River

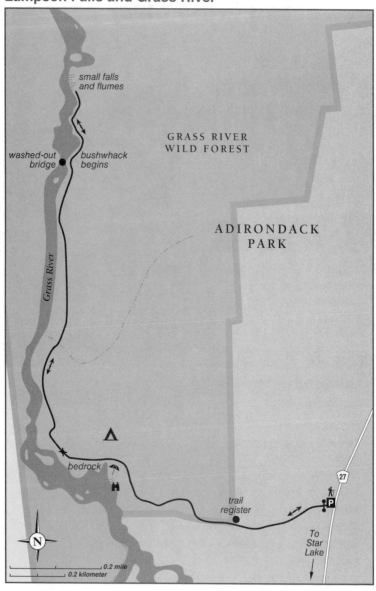

small falls and flumes

GRASS RIVER WILD FOREST

washed-out bridge

bushwhack begins

ADIRONDACK PARK

Grass River

bedrock

trail register

27

To Star Lake

N

0.2 mile

0.2 kilometer

Overview

As one of a few hikes with sections that are wheelchair accessible, this trail is ideal for families with limited mobility or who just prefer a trip that does not require constant weaving around obstacles. If you prefer obstacles, you can always extend your trip to include the riverside trail and a little extra bushwhacking downstream to explore some interesting cataracts and flumes. Lampson Falls is also a popular swimming spot during the summer, but if you continue along the riverside trail, you will find solitude.

Route Details

Parking for the trailhead is parallel to County Road 27; two of the five designated spaces are reserved for handicapped parking, though an additional car or two could fit in behind the regular parking spaces. The trail begins at the southern end of the pullout, past a vehicle barrier. The trail is actually a crushed-gravel access road, which is why it is designated universally accessible. The trail register and a map of the trail system are located a little less than 0.3 mile past the vehicle barrier. The forest is a mixture of eastern white pines and hardwoods with a lush and thick understory of ferns. The terrain,

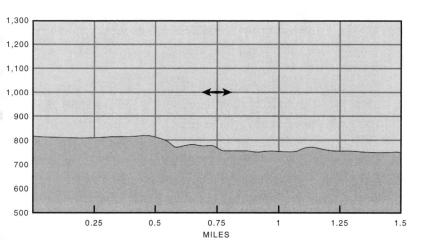

befitting a wheelchair-accessible trail, is exceptionally flat, and you will hear the roar of the falls long before you reach the wheelchair-accessible viewing area. Follow the wide path through a series of switchbacks and numerous turning points, constructed out of landscape timbers and filled with gravel, to the viewing spot above the falls. From the top of the falls, it is easy to see why this is a popular attraction, as the Grass River cascades down over the exposed bedrock in a frothy torrent. From this vantage point, keep an eye out for the swifts that swoop and dive as they ride updrafts and feast on insects caught above the falls. To reach the base of the falls, you can choose any number of footpaths or scramble down the rocks, but the accessible portion of the trail ends here.

At the base of the falls is a sandy beach that is an obvious congregation point and an unfortunate reminder that not all people follow the Department of Environmental Conservation's carry-in, carry-out policy. This is an easy place to implement one of my preferred policies: carry in, carry one more out. From the sandy beach, you can scramble up a steep hillside to reach exposed portions of bedrock directly across from the waterfall. This is my favorite vantage point of the falls and is an excellent spot to stop and enjoy the view. Back among the tall pines is a designated camping area that includes the standard pit toilet but offers no views of the waterfall or river. Continue along the bedrock, across from the falls, to a rocky peninsula for another picnicking spot, as well as the beginning of the riverside trail.

The trail was in serious disrepair in 2009, with multiple areas of nearly impassable blowdown. However, Department of Environmental Conservation and volunteer trail crews clear blowdown regularly, so the trail may have been returned to a suitable condition, making it an easy riverside stroll. Marked with red disks, the trail is evidently rarely used, and thick overgrown vegetation on either side masks the conditions underfoot. Brambles are a significant part of the overgrowth, so gaiters are recommended during the summer.

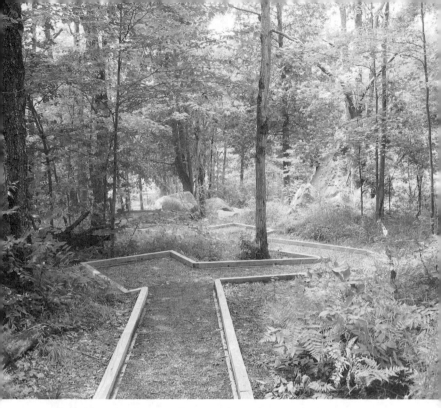

ACCESSIBLE TRAIL TO LAMPSON FALLS

Additionally, numerous beaver-plunge holes are hidden by the dense overgrowth, so use caution when you cannot see your footing.

In sharp contrast to the turbulent falls, the river seems almost placid, and its grass- and fern-lined banks make for a tranquil setting. At 1.5 miles the trail intersects an overgrown road to your right, and the remnants of a foundation are visible on both banks. Readers of the old trail guides will discover that the bridge connecting the two banks was washed out in 1998 and has not been replaced. The foundations sit on either side of a small flume, where the river narrows from dozens of feet to just a few feet. This is the formal end of the trail, which is unfortunate because several flumes, falls, and cataracts farther downstream add great interest to the trip. To see these spectacles, you will have to follow old footpaths and bushwhack a bit, but rest assured, other hikers have been here before, so the path is distinct most of the way. Over the next 0.3 mile, the placid waters transform into frothing cascades as the river drops quickly and the lush, wide banks constrict to rocky ledges. You will see multiple flumes and falls along the paths, but my favorite is where the river forks at a tiny, rocky island. The eastern fork drops vertically to form a narrow waterfall, after which the flow diminishes into slack water, while the western leg forms a frothing cataract. You can reach the island by crossing above the tiny waterfall or rock-hopping in the slack water. This section of the river coincides with the disappearance of the old footpaths and makes a good end for the river exploration.

Directions

From the intersection of NY 3 and Youngs Road in Star Lake, head 6.3 miles northwest along NY 3, and turn right onto CR 27/CR 27A. Continue 0.8 mile, and turn right onto CR 27/Degrasse-Fine Road heading north. Follow CR 27 north 7.8 miles, and turn right to stay on CR 27, now also known as Fine-Canton-Lisbon Road. Continue on CR 27 another 4.5 miles, passing the airstrip along the way. The parking area will be on your left.

Floodwood

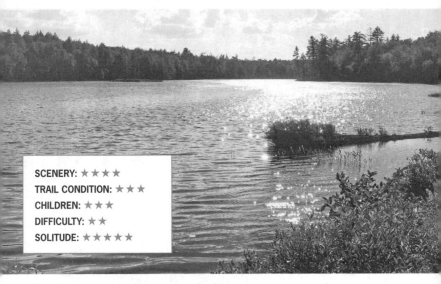

SCENERY: ★ ★ ★ ★
TRAIL CONDITION: ★ ★ ★
CHILDREN: ★ ★ ★
DIFFICULTY: ★ ★
SOLITUDE: ★ ★ ★ ★ ★

MIDDLE POND SEEN FROM FLOODWOOD ROAD

GPS COORDINATES: N44° 18.497'   W74° 21.550'

DISTANCE & CONFIGURATION: 8.5-mile loop

HIKING TIME: 3–4 hours

HIGHLIGHTS: Multiple ponds

ELEVATION: 1,590' at trailhead, with no significant rise along the trail

ACCESS: $8 day-use fee during camping season; free when camping at Fish Creek Pond/ Rollins Pond Campgrounds or with an Empire Passport. Campgrounds open mid-April–late-October; check the Department of Environmental Conservation campground schedule for exact dates: www.dec.ny.gov/outdoor/7820.html.

MAPS: National Geographic *Adirondack Park, Saranac/Paul Smiths* (#746)

FACILITIES: Restrooms, swimming beach, boat rentals when campgrounds are open

WHEELCHAIR ACCESS: No

COMMENTS: Access is allowed and the day-use fee is waived during the off-season, but hikers will have to hike in along the access road from NY 30, which adds 0.8 mile to the trip. Campground roads are not plowed during the winter.

CONTACTS: Fish Creek Pond Campground: www.dec.ny.gov/outdoor/24466.html; Northern Adirondacks trail information: www.dec.ny.gov/outdoor/9196.html; emergency contact: 518-891-0235

Floodwood

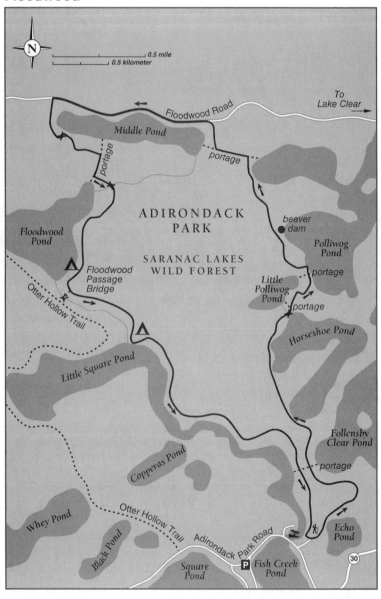

Overview

At first glance, this hike may seem long, but the gently rolling terrain makes it an easy and relatively quick hike. Winding through a hardwood forest, the trail leads you from one pristine pond to another, offering scenery and solitude the whole trip. Though the trail starts and ends in a bustling campground, it is likely that the only people you will encounter are canoeists at the numerous portages that crisscross the trail.

Route Details

The trailhead is slightly different from the other Adirondack trailheads in that access is through a campground, which includes a day-use fee of $8; no designated parking is located immediately nearby; and there is no trail register. The fee is waived if you are camping at either Fish Creek Pond or Rollins Pond Campgrounds; for a description of the latter, see *Best Tent Camping: New York State*. The parking areas closest to the trailhead are in the day-use area near the swimming beach (go left after the registration booth) or near the basketball courts, the recreation area, and campsite 50, past the boat launch area (go right after the registration booth). Make sure to

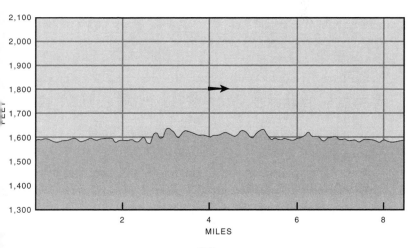

grab a campground map, as it makes finding the trailhead easier and includes a trail map.

The trailhead is located on the access road for Fish Creek Pond campsites C1–C7. While walking up the road, you will see red Department of Environmental Conservation snowmobile trail markers and will come upon two log stumps that act as vehicle barriers on your right. You can begin here or farther up the road, near campsite C7. The trail description included here is from the vehicle barrier heading north along the eastern leg and returning south along the western leg. There is little difference heading clockwise or counterclockwise, though if you plan to walk only one leg of the trip, then I would choose the western leg, as it is in better shape and a flooded area on the eastern leg may seem impassable.

The trail winds north under a canopy of tall pines as well as multiple species of birch, and within a few hundred yards you will catch glimpses of Echo Pond. Dense pine saplings quickly dampen the noise from the campground, and you feel removed and remote. Another element you will notice is that the trail is basically flat, and your pace will be closer to walking along a sidewalk than hiking. Trail markers switch between snowmobile and foot-trail disks, but the path is so distinct that very little marking is necessary. You will catch glimpses of the much larger Follensby Clear Pond to your right and quickly come to a distinct intersection at mile 0.7. The east–west trail that bisects the hiking trail is the first of several canoe carries and provides a portage from Fish Creek Pond to Follensby Clear Pond. You will cross this portage again on the return trip, but for now it provides a convenient way to get an up close view of the pond to the west. The more heavily trodden canoe carry reveals that canoeing is the dominant activity in the area, which provides the hiker a bit more solitude on the trail.

Continuing straight ahead, you will notice that the hemlocks and birches are quite large and tower overhead. Deep views into the forest contrast with limited views out onto the bodies of water, as hemlock saplings crowd the shorelines. You first encounter

Horseshoe Pond and walk along its edge through thicker hemlocks 1 mile from the start. At 1.4 miles, you come to a large moss-covered, mucky area that is the beginning of a spruce swamp bisected by the trail. At 1.8 miles it may seem like you are coming up on another pond, but it is the opposite leg of Horseshoe Pond. The shore is distinctly more visible to your right as you head more directly north. At 2.3 miles, you come to the outlet of Little Polliwog Pond as it empties into Horseshoe Pond. A sign warns that the bridge is out; indeed, the bridge has fallen apart, though remnants of rickety boards laid on logs provide a zigzag crossing. On the other side, the trail briefly shares the canoe carry between Little Polliwog and Horseshoe Ponds. At mile 2.9 you come across the canoe carry between Little Polliwog and Polliwog Ponds through a stand of hemlocks.

Around 3 miles you arrive at a broad, flooded section of the trail created by a recently constructed beaver dam. At this point your options for crossing the flooded section are limited. Crossing on top of the dam will likely be your driest option, but don't count on having dry feet afterward. The trail on the other side is less clear and is overgrown, and trail markers seemed to be missing when I was there. However, though the trail appears to be more of a herd path, it does continue through a couple of muddy areas, and red trail markers are visible again in less than 0.3 mile. You pass by another bay of Polliwog Pond at 3.2 miles, and at 3.4 miles you come to a T in the path. Signs indicate that the snowmobile trail continues to your left. The path joining the trail from your right is the canoe carry between Polliwog Pond and Middle Pond. Head west (left) along the combined trail and portage less than 0.3 mile, where the portage continues straight and the trail veers right toward Floodwood Road. Less than 0.1 mile ahead is Floodwood Road, which you will follow 1 mile west to pick up the western leg of the loop. It might seem odd to include a road with a trail, but the road is actually a pleasant variation on the trip. This seldom-used dirt road passes within feet of Middle Pond, and because it is free of roots and other obstructions, you can spend the mile looking out on the placid waters of the

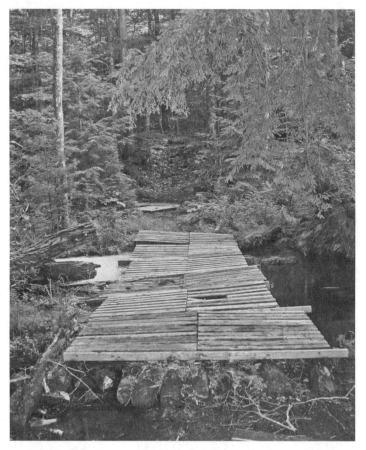

WOOD PALLETS ACROSS AN INLET OF FLOODWOOD POND SERVE AS A BRIDGE.

pond. You will pass one of several designated primitive campsites along the road.

At 4.7 miles you pick the trail up again and head back into the woods along a ridge that sits above Middle Pond. In less than 0.3 mile the trail heads east, and you cross a log bridge. You will have left the shores of Middle Pond by now, but you have another chance to return to its shores at 5.1 miles, when you arrive at a fork in the trail.

Continuing south along the trail, you catch glimpses of Floodwood Pond just before you reach yet another fork; the path ahead leads to the pond's shores, while the trail continues on your left. Pallets laid in pairs form a bridge across a stream, the outlet of Middle Pond into Floodwood Pond, at 5.4 miles. Shortly after the crossing, you come back to Floodwood Pond and stroll along its shores for the next 0.5 mile. At 6 miles, you pass through a designated campsite near where Floodwood Pond flows into a creek. Take a left at the campsite, and briefly head west, where you reach another fork in the trail. To the right are Floodwood Passage Bridge and Otter Hollow Trail; these take you back to the campgrounds, while the Floodwood Trail continues straight ahead beside the creek. Follow the Floodwood Trail as it climbs slightly alongside the creek and then descends around 6.5 miles to another designated campsite. These designated campsites are used by canoeists and kayakers, but if they are vacant, their picnic tables make an excellent spot to stop, sit, and enjoy the scenery. The trail turns left at the campsite and continues along the shore of Little Square Pond through a couple more designated campsites.

The trail continues southeast along Little Square Pond as it transitions into Fish Creek Pond. From this point on, the trail delves deeper into the forest, and views of the water are limited to occasional glimpses. At mile 8 you pass the first canoe carry you encountered near the beginning and quickly come to the end of the trail at campsite C7.

Directions

From Tupper Lake, head east on NY 3/NY 30. At 5.3 miles, turn left to stay on NY 30. After another 5.4 miles, turn left at the main entrance to the Fish Creek Pond and Rollins Pond Campgrounds. You will have to pay a day-use fee of $8 unless you are camping at either campground. The main parking area is to the left of the registration booth. The trailhead is along the access road to campsites C1–C7.

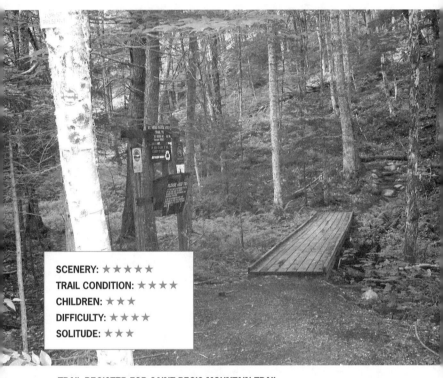

SCENERY: ★ ★ ★ ★ ★
TRAIL CONDITION: ★ ★ ★ ★
CHILDREN: ★ ★ ★
DIFFICULTY: ★ ★ ★ ★
SOLITUDE: ★ ★ ★

TRAIL REGISTER FOR SAINT REGIS MOUNTAIN TRAIL

GPS COORDINATES: N44° 25.826'   W74° 17.950'

DISTANCE & CONFIGURATION: 6.7-mile out-and-back

HIKING TIME: 3–4 hours

HIGHLIGHTS: Panoramic views, fire tower

ELEVATION: 1,622' at trailhead, 2,874' at highest point

ACCESS: Open 24/7; no fees or permits required

MAPS: National Geographic *Adirondack Park, Saranac/Paul Smiths* (#746)

FACILITIES: None

WHEELCHAIR ACCESS: No

CONTACTS: Northern Adirondack trail information: www.dec.ny.gov/outdoor/9196.html; emergency contact: 518-891-0235

Overview

Best known for its mostly flat terrain, the northern section of the Adirondacks has many excellent extended canoe trips. Most notable is the Saint Regis Canoe Area. However, looming over this area of hundreds of ponds, lakes, and interconnected waterways is Saint Regis Mountain. For a truly majestic view, its summit is unsurpassed.

Route Details

The actual trailhead is a short distance south of the large and well-maintained parking area. From the parking area, no signs point you to the trail. To reach it, head south down Topridge Road across the Saint Regis River, whose rushing waters you probably noticed as soon as you parked. Approximately 0.1 mile down the road, you will see the trail register just off to the right. Next to the register is a finely built log-and-plank bridge that is indicative of ongoing work to maintain the trail. Indeed, the presence of so many mucky areas, despite the amount of maintenance, shows how popular this trail is. The Department of Environmental Conservation (DEC) constructed the bridge when it rerouted the trail in 1999, but forestry students from Paul Smith's College and stewards have done much of the work evident throughout. Anyone wishing for solitude atop the mountain would be wise to follow a few rules of thumb: First, hike during the week rather than on weekends, and especially avoid holiday weekends. Second, hike when school is in session. Last, start earlier, which usually ensures you some time to yourself at the peak and other destinations where hikers typically congregate.

The trail, marked with red disks, follows generally rolling terrain through mature hardwoods dotted with large hemlocks. Approximately 0.3 mile in, you will pass a sheer rock face covered in moss and ferns. This adds some variation to the hike, but the dominant feature before the summit is the deep forest. At 1 mile, you will walk over a small hillock heavily shaded by hemlocks and then descend briefly back into the mixed hardwood forest. The trail becomes very

Saint Regis Mountain

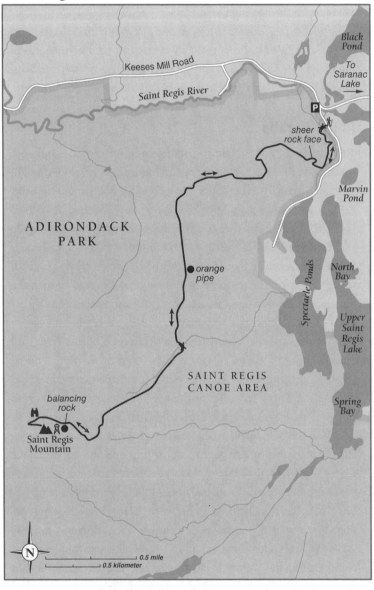

straight and begins to climb afterward, but the grade is gradual and almost difficult to notice. You pass an orange-painted pipe surrounded by stones on the left at 1.7 miles; this is approximately the halfway point of the trail. After a slight descent around mile 2.1, you come to a fork and a bridge that crosses a small stream. The trail to your left is the old trail that is no longer maintained.

Once you cross the bridge, the ascent to the summit truly begins. Gradual at first, it becomes much steeper as you near the summit. The stream you crossed flows on your right as you climb and occasionally flows over the trail nearer the summit. Stone steps built along the trail help prevent further erosion, but long sections of muddy areas become inevitable. Indeed, the trail has been worn into a rut more than a foot deep. Estimating how far along the trail these mires are is futile, as one slick seems to grow larger than the previous one, and you quickly lose track of how many you cross. At 2.9 miles, you pass a vertical rock face almost entirely covered in moss. Another distinct landmark is at mile 3.1, where you pass a large balancing rock on your left and another boulder directly to your right. Passage between these boulders is essentially the last portion of steep climbing, and the final elevation gains are over flatter portions. Winding

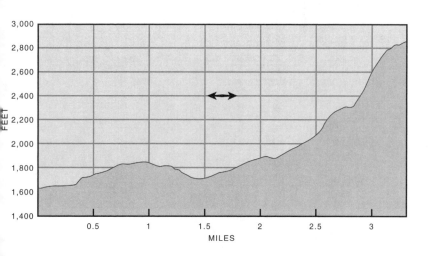

around the contours of the peak, the trail is shaded by mostly paper birches with an occasional mountain ash. Keep an eye out on your right for a lookout, which offers good panoramic views and a glimpse of the fire tower.

At the summit, you have 360-degree views of the myriad lakes and ponds nestled among forested hills and small mountains within the immediate vicinity, with the High Peaks towering off to the south. The fire tower has gone through renovation by the DEC, Student Conservation Association Adirondack AmeriCorps Program, and Friends of St. Regis Mountain Fire Tower. The restoration of the fire tower is complete, and the tower is now publicly accessible. Its location in a canoe area had been a much-debated issue. The DEC Master Plan calls for the removal of fire towers from wild forest areas, which include canoe areas, but revisions and conflicts with the New York Historic Preservation Act of 1980 complicate the matter. Many groups have formed to protect and restore fire towers on this and other peaks, claiming that fire towers are part of the region's history and that their stewards were instrumental in educating the public and helping to protect and preserve the wilderness.

Directions

From Tupper Lake, head east on NY 3/NY 30. Turn left to stay on NY 30 at 5.3 miles. At 14.2 more miles turn left again to stay on NY 30. Turn left onto Keeses Mill Road at 6.9 miles. The DEC parking area is 2.6 miles ahead on the left.

36

Debar Mountain

SCENERY: ★ ★ ★ ★
TRAIL CONDITION: ★ ★ ★ ★ ★
CHILDREN: ★ ★
DIFFICULTY: ★ ★ ★ ★
SOLITUDE: ★ ★ ★

SCENE ATOP DEBAR MOUNTAIN

GPS COORDINATES: N44° 34.639'   W74° 16.735'

DISTANCE & CONFIGURATION: 8.8-mile out-and-back, 7.4-mile out-and-back from trail-head parking area (seasonal)

HIKING TIME: 4.5–5.5 hours

HIGHLIGHTS: Panoramic views, Bald Peak, old foundation

ELEVATION: 1,564' at trailhead, 3,305' at Debar Mountain peak

ACCESS: $8 day-use fee during camping season; free when camping at Meacham Lake Campground or with an Empire Passport. Campground open mid-May–mid-October; check the Department of Environmental Conservation campground schedule for exact dates: www. dec.ny.gov/outdoor/7820.html.

MAPS: National Geographic *Adirondack Park, Saranac/Paul Smiths* (#746)

FACILITIES: Restrooms, swimming beach, boat rentals when campgrounds are open

WHEELCHAIR ACCESS: No

COMMENTS: Access is allowed and the day-use fee is waived during the off-season, but you will have to hike in along the access road from NY 30, which adds 2 miles to the trip. Campground roads are not plowed during the winter. The final 0.25-mile section to the peak will likely require crampons and an ice ax in winter.

CONTACTS: Meacham Lake Campground: www.dec.ny.gov/outdoor/24481.html; Northern Adirondack trail information: www.dec.ny.gov/outdoor/9196.html; emergency contact: 518-891-0235

Debar Mountain

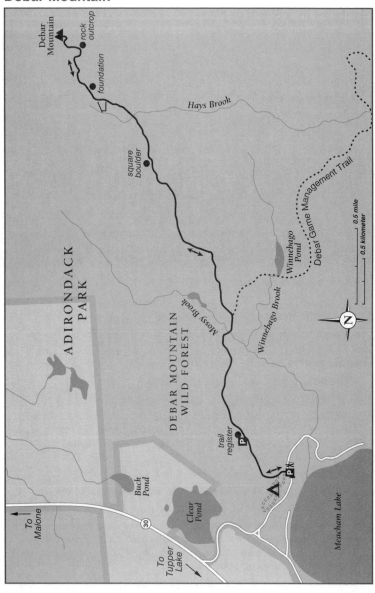

Overview

Like many peak trails in the Adirondacks, this trail begins along level terrain but quickly steepens as you approach the summit. Near the peak, the trail is particularly steep—near vertical in some sections—and will require use of your hands in some sections. But the climb is worth it, and you will be rewarded with a sprawling panorama of the Northern Adirondacks.

Route Details

The first decision you will have to make is whether to park in the public parking area located near the beach or at the trailhead parking area, via the access road. The distance from the public parking area to the end of the access road is roughly 0.7 mile, so parking at its end will reduce the trip by about a 1.4 miles overall. The road is in good condition, so most vehicles with have little trouble along the flat drive. But it is a seasonal road and may be closed, so plan your trip to include the access road just in case. Directions and mileage given here include the access road.

From the parking area in front of the Meacham Lake Recreation Field (near campsites 45–47), head north away from the beach

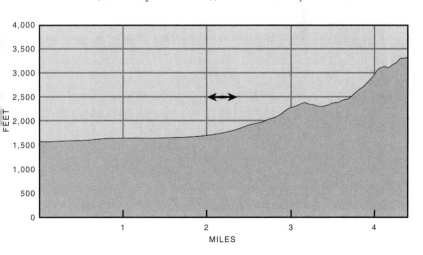

to the main campsite road. Follow this road east a short distance, and take the first left, near campsite 48. Continue north along the road past campsite 37 to a vehicle-barrier gate and the start of the access road; signs indicate this is the TRAIL TO DEBAR. The access road is flat and wide and meanders north another 0.5 mile to the trailhead, second parking area, and trail register.

The second parking area is a large pulloff on the north side of the road, a short distance before another vehicle-barrier gate and the trail register. Past the barrier gate, the trail still follows an old road, but its closure to regular vehicle traffic has allowed nature to encroach back on the road, transforming the route into a nice broad footpath. With a sandy base and moss- and grass-lined shoulders, the path is quite an easy and pleasant stroll following a mostly level course. The trail weaves between a single- and doubletrack, and two hikers could walk side by side much of the way. You will cross a mossy brook, a tributary to Winnebago Brook, a little over 0.75 mile past the trail register. Less than 0.25 mile farther, 1.6 miles overall, is the intersection with the main trail to Debar Mountain on your left. Straight ahead, the Debar Game Management Trail continues past Debar Meadows, 5 miles, to County Road 26, 6.3 miles.

Turn left (north) onto the main Debar Mountain trail. The trail is sporadically marked with red and yellow trail disks, but they are so infrequent that they are not as reliable as the path worn by the many previous hikers. The trail narrows from here forward, with the grade growing steadily steeper as you begin the 1,700-foot ascent to the peak. The first ascent (roughly 700 feet over the next 1.5 miles) culminates at the saddle between Black Peak to the north and an unnamed knob to the south. Along the first part of this ascent, you will pass a log-and-plank bridge over a seasonal stream, shortly followed by a large, square boulder that interrupts the trail about three-quarters of the way up. At the saddle, the trail levels off and then dips down to cross Hays Brook, after which the climbing begins again.

From the brook crossing, another 1.1 miles and roughly 1,000 feet of ascent remain. In less than 0.25 mile, pass the Debar Mountain

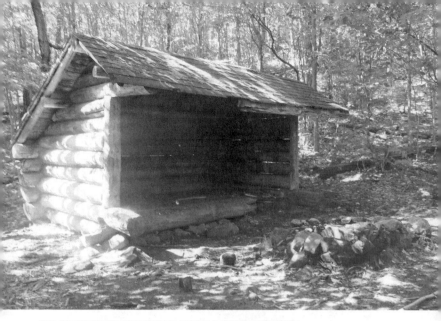

THE DEBAR MOUNTAIN LEAN-TO MAKES A GREAT REST STOP.

Lean-To on the left. A little over 0.1 mile ahead, pass through a clearing along the trail. Look to your right and you will find the remains of the fire tower cabin foundation.

Past the clearing, the grade begins to steepen even more, and you may find you need your hands to negotiate some of the steeper sections. A half mile later and 650 feet higher, you reach a recent slide that looms over the trail, 4.1 miles overall. At first glance it appears that the trail passes beneath this imposing and nearly vertical outcrop of rock, but the trail actually ascends to its left. If you didn't need to use your hands to assist your climb before, you surely will now. Water flows freely through the vertical jumble of rocks and roots, making choosing your footing especially tricky at times. In winter this portion may be impassable for those who did not bring crampons or an ice ax. (Remember, winter in the Adirondacks can start as early as late September and continue into early May.) It is another 0.25 mile and roughly 200 feet to the peak.

The trail levels off briefly before you reach the actual summit. There may be a bit of confusion as to how to best reach it as dense spruce surrounds the bald peak. You can either scramble up a short

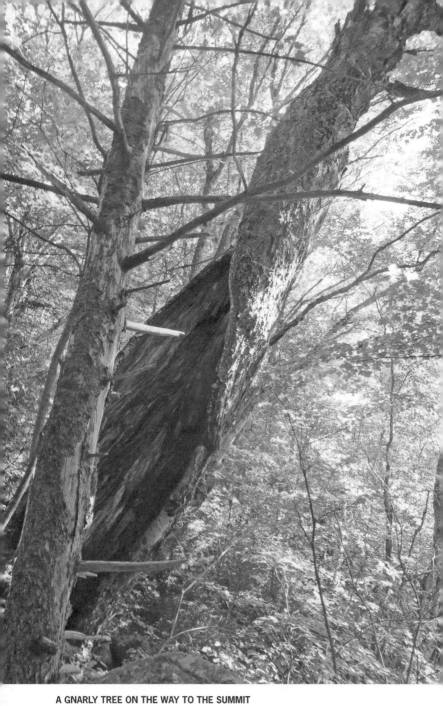

A GNARLY TREE ON THE WAY TO THE SUMMIT

rock face on the left or continue onto the north side of the peak and double back, pushing your way through the dense evergreens. Either way, what awaits is a sprawling panorama of the Northern Adirondacks. From the peak, you are looking back southwest onto Meacham Lake and Clear Pond and can practically trace the path you traversed. Also atop the bald peak are the remains of the old fire tower foundation and anchor points. Return the way you came, taking your time descending the vertical portions for a round-trip of 8.8 miles.

Directions

From Tupper Lake, head east on NY 3/NY 30. At 5.3 miles, turn left to head north on NY 30. After 14.2 more miles turn left to remain on NY 30. Follow NY 30 another 18.5 miles north, and the entrance to the Meacham Lake State Campground will be on the right. Follow Meacham Road to the campground entrance, 0.6 mile, and turn left. Continue another 0.5 mile to the main parking area, a short distance east past the registration both.

High Peaks (Hikes 37–46)

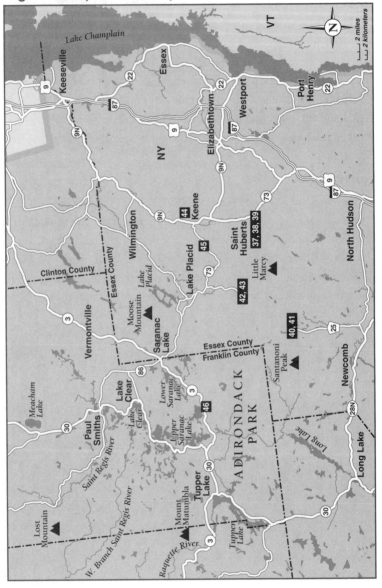

High Peaks

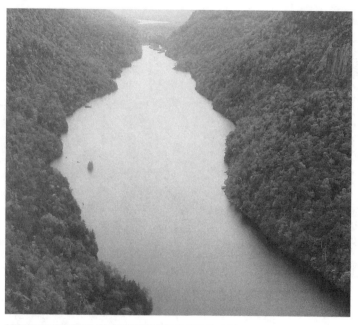

AUSABLE LAKE SEEN FROM FISH HAWK CLIFFS (Trail 38, Ausable River: East River Trail, page 262)

37

Ausable River:
West River Trail

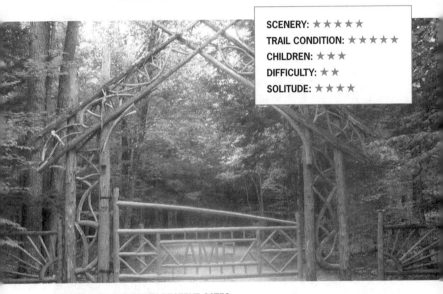

SCENERY: ★ ★ ★ ★ ★
TRAIL CONDITION: ★ ★ ★ ★ ★
CHILDREN: ★ ★ ★
DIFFICULTY: ★ ★
SOLITUDE: ★ ★ ★ ★

ADIRONDACK MOUNTAIN RESERVE GATES

GPS COORDINATES: Parking area: N44° 08.986'   W73° 46.075'
Trailhead: N44° 08.992'   W73° 46.843'

DISTANCE & CONFIGURATION: 10.8-mile out-and-back or 9.7-mile loop if combined with
Ausable River: East River Trail (see page 262)

HIKING TIME: 3–4 hours one-way

HIGHLIGHTS: Spectacular waterfalls, scenic lookout, riverside stroll

ELEVATION: 1,266' at trailhead, 2,493' at highest point

ACCESS: Open 24/7; no fees or permits required. Guests must register at the gatehouse.

MAPS: Adirondack Mountain Reserve map: tinyurl.com/adkmtnreserve; National Geographic *Adirondack Park, Lake Placid/High Peaks* (#742)

FACILITIES: None

WHEELCHAIR ACCESS: No

COMMENTS: This trail is on private property, but access to the public is granted through
an easement. However, special rules apply; these are briefly described on the following
pages and available on the Department of Environmental Conservation website (below).

CONTACTS: Adirondack Mountain Reserve: www.dec.ny.gov/lands/100916.html; emergency contact: 518-891-0235

Overview

The East Branch of Ausable (pronounced "aw-say-bull") River is a smorgasbord of waterfalls. From mossy cascades and powerful flumes to misty veils and thunderous sheer drops, the variety and multitude of waterfalls make this an ideal hike for waterfall lovers. The hike is rich with scenic lookouts and riverside strolling—overall an excellent excursion.

Route Details

The trail lies entirely within the property lines of the Adirondack Mountain Reserve (AMR), so hikers should be aware of several restrictions. The rules are strictly enforced and posted when entering the property. The main restrictions are that pets are not allowed, and no firearms, camping, hunting, fishing, swimming, or boating is allowed. Additionally, off-trail travel, bushwhacking, and rock climbing are prohibited. Despite the restrictions, one major advantage of the trail's being on private property is its superb condition. There are few muddy areas, trails are clear of blowdown, and bridges are all in great condition. Parking is approximately 0.7 mile from the trailhead and register but is included in the mileage given.

The large parking area near NY 73 can accommodate dozens of cars, so finding a spot should be straightforward. Head west along Ausable Club Road. At a little more than 0.1 mile, you pass the trailhead for Round and Dix Mountains. Roughly 0.3 mile later, you pass a second trailhead junction, Stimson Trail, as well as a golf course. Just past the tennis courts, you will see a large lime-green building and reach Lake Road at 0.6 mile. Turn left down the road, and head past several small cabins to the AMR trail register. All hikers must sign in and out at the register. Continue down the road past the ornate wooden gate. A gabled arch, constructed from round and irregular logs and branches, vaults the gate, which is constructed similarly and has AMR built into its center. The gate was reconstructed in 1986 as part of the AMR's centennial observances and is a replica of the original.

Ausable River: West River Trail

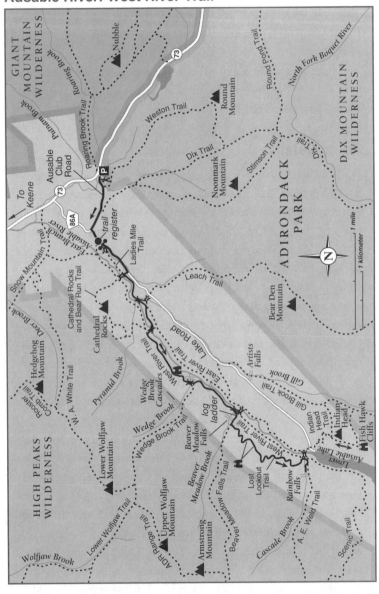

Shortly after the gate, you pass Ladies Mile Trail, which, if you want to get off the club's road sooner, also leads to West River Trail. A second intersection with Ladies Mile Trail is 0.3 mile past the gate, 1 mile total. This junction connects to West River Trail directly, but yards ahead is a junction with East River Trail (an alternate way to reach West River Trail) and likely your return trip if you make the complete loop. Cross the wooden plank bridge, and head 0.3 mile west to another trail junction. Straight ahead are East River Trail and the path back to Lake Road, while Bear Run, Cathedral Rocks, and West River Trails are off to the right. Cross the bridge over the East Branch of Ausable River, and turn left onto the trail. West River Trail, marked with yellow markers, heads west, while Bear Run and Cathedral Rocks Trails, marked in red, head north.

The trail heads west under towering hemlocks and climbs gradually above the river gorge. At times you hike close to the river, but you veer away into the surrounding forest over many sections. Grades are gentle, and at 1.7 miles, you cross Pyramid Brook, after which the trail heads back toward the river. At 1.8 miles, you reconnect with Bear Run, Cathedral Rocks, and Pyramid Brook Trails. Approximately 0.1 mile ahead, you reach another junction and a

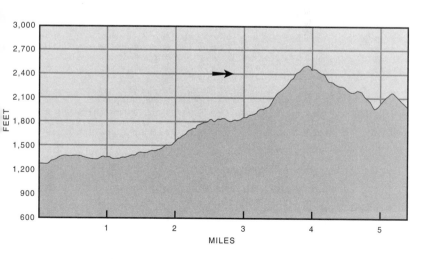

green trail sign indicating East River Trail, Lake Road, and Canyon Bridge to your left; West River Trail and Wolfjaw straight ahead; and Bear Run, Cathedral Rocks, and West River Trails back the way you came. The trail climbs a bit past this intersection, and the drop down to the river is significant at this point. You can see small cascades and flumes along the river, and the roaring of the water drowns out most sounds. The sounds and views decrease as you climb away from the river for the next 0.5 mile, but you soon return; at 2.4 miles you come across a lookout to a waterfall along the river. This lookout is to the left of the trail, and there is a precipitous drop, so take care while viewing the waterfall. Shortly after, the trail swings north to follow a feeder brook, Wedge Brook, a short distance and then crosses the brook over a bridge. The bridge spans the brook between two waterfalls. The lower is really a small cascade, and the second is a small waterfall that branches around a large rock and tumbles into a pool above the bridge. On the other side is Wedge Brook Trail to Lower Wolfjaw, and a sign indicates that the Wedge Brook Cascades are a couple hundred yards away. A short climb along this trail reveals a series of small cascades that weave their way down mossy crevices in the rock to the small pool below.

Back along the main trail, you reach the river in less than 0.3 mile, and you will notice that it is now surging through tight flumes and small cascades at many points. At 2.9 miles, you see another waterfall, which is approximately 25 feet high, with a very powerful surge of water that spurts out nearly horizontally as the river is restricted to a few feet through the narrow gorge. Occasional vantage points are available, but take care when trying to view this fall, as the river gorge is very steep and treacherous. After this waterfall, the river levels off and spreads out among the boulders, but many tiny falls and cascades remain throughout.

At 3.3 miles, the trail reaches a small brook and turns north, almost immediately after which you reach Beaver Meadow Falls. Unlike the last falls, which fell in a powerful surge, Beaver Meadow Falls is almost like a light rain or mist. Often referred to as a bridal-veil

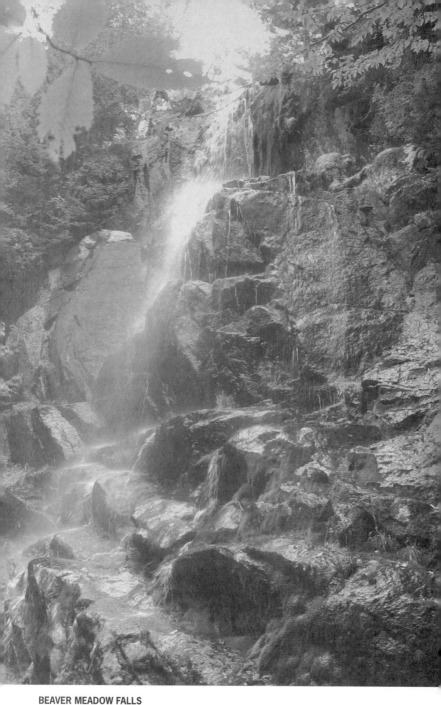

BEAVER MEADOW FALLS

falls, Beaver Meadow Falls is about 60 feet high. A bridge that spans the brook provides a great place to admire and photograph the falls.

West River Trail continues along the river west through some marshy sections and slow-flowing waters that add variety and interest. However, a side trip along Lost Lookout Trail provides an inspiring view of Lower Ausable Lake and a particularly interesting view of Rainbow Falls.

To reach the Lost Lookout Trail, climb the log ladder on the other side of Beaver Meadow Falls. As you climb alongside Beaver Meadow Falls, you can see its entirety. The trail, marked in blue, leads to Gothics and Armstrong Mountains and climbs fairly steeply. You quickly reach the Lost Lookout fork on your left, which is marked in red disks and is 0.2 mile from Beaver Meadow Falls, 3.5 miles from the start. The trail climbs steadily through the beech-and-maple forest another 0.3 mile, where you reach the first of two lookouts. You can see Lower Ausable Lake, Indian Head, and Fish Hawk Cliffs nearby, as well as Bear Den, Dial, and Nippletop Mountains, among other peaks to the south. The second lookout is nearby and offers the same views after you traverse a short but steep descent. The trail continues southwest and descends for the next 0.8 mile. You will begin to hear the deep roar of Rainbow Falls and soon glimpse the 150-foot waterfall. Extremely sheer drop-offs are beside the trail, so do not attempt to climb down to get to the falls from here. A separate trail farther ahead brings you to the base of Rainbow Falls. The trail winds down steeply for the next 0.3 mile, after which you reach the intersection with West River Trail. The trail, marked in yellow, quickly leads to a dam that marks the end of Lower Ausable Lake and the head of the East Branch of Ausable River. After crossing Cascade Brook, you reach a long log-and-plank bridge that crosses the river below this dam and leads to East River Trail, as well as Indian Head and Fish Hawk Cliffs on the left. A trail to the right leads to Sawteeth and Gothics Mountains, as well as Rainbow Falls. You will return to this point, 4.9 miles from the start, so that you can head back along East River Trail.

Before returning, take the blue-marked trail to the right to see these spectacular falls, less than 0.3 mile away. Shortly after beginning along the blue trail, you reach a fork with a yellow-marked trail that indicates Sawteeth Mountain (via the scenic route) on the left and Gothics Mountain, Sawteeth Mountain (presumably along a hideous stretch of trail), and Rainbow Falls off to the right on the blue trail. A few hundred feet later, the trail to Gothics and the others, marked in blue, diverges to the left, while the path to the falls continues to your right but is now marked sporadically in red. You will pass several pipes, both plastic and steel, as you weave your way through boulders to the base of the sheer cliffs that form the falls. A sheer rock wall forms on your left as you work your way up alongside Cascade Brook to the base of Rainbow Falls. The canyon formed by the sheer rock walls amplifies the thundering of the falls as the water drops 150 feet. Mist sprayed on the opposite wall provides a haven for moss, while the water has scoured clean the rock wall on the waterfall side. The contrast of verdant green and jet black on the opposing walls is a unique scene that invites lingering. Head back to the dam to reach East River Trail as well as the spectacular views from Indian Head and Fish Hawk Cliffs.

Directions

From I-87, take Exit 30 for US 9, and head north. Go 2.2 miles on US 9, and make a slight left onto NY 73. In 5.4 miles look for Ausable Club Road on your left just after descending a steep hill.

From the intersection of NY 9N and NY 73, head southeast on NY 73. In 6.1 miles, Ausable Club Road is on your right, directly across from the Giant Mountain parking area, described on page 276. The parking area is almost immediately on your left after you turn onto Ausable Club Road.

Ausable River:
East River Trail

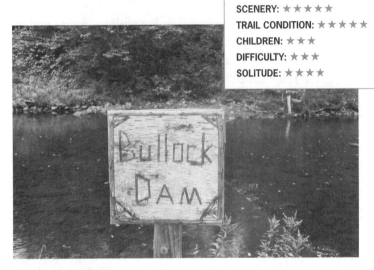

SIGN AT BULLOCK DAM

GPS COORDINATES: Parking area: N44° 08.986' W73° 46.075'
Trailhead: N44° 08.992' W73° 46.843'

DISTANCE & CONFIGURATION: 9.7-mile loop if combined with Ausable River: West River Trail (see page 254), or 8.6-mile out-and-back, plus 1.6-mile out-and-back side trip to Indian Head and Fish Hawk Cliffs

HIKING TIME: 3–4 hours one-way

HIGHLIGHTS: Scenic views, dramatic cliffs, spectacular waterfall, riverside stroll

ELEVATION: 1,960' at trailhead, 2,657' at highest point (on side trip)

ACCESS: Open 24/7; no fees or permits required. Guests must register at the gatehouse.

MAPS: Adirondack Mountain Reserve map: tinyurl.com/adkmtnreserve; National Geographic *Adirondack Park, Lake Placid/High Peaks* (#742)

FACILITIES: None

WHEELCHAIR ACCESS: No

COMMENTS: This trail is on private property, but access to the public is granted through an easement. However, special rules apply; these are briefly described on the following pages and available on the Department of Environmental Conservation website (below).

CONTACTS: Adirondack Mountain Reserve: www.dec.ny.gov/lands/100916.html; emergency contact: 518-891-0235

Overview

East River Trail is the return leg of a loop along the East Branch of Ausable (pronounced "aw-say-bull") River. This section has fewer waterfalls, but it does include a side trip to Indian Head and Fish Hawk Cliffs, which have impressive views and dramatic scenery of their own.

Route Details

You can hike the east section of Ausable River on its own, but I found it to be an excellent return trip for West River Trail (described on page 254). A side trip to Indian Head and Fish Hawk Cliffs reveals amazing views and is well worth the extra 1.6 miles. Directions back to the parking area along NY 73 and for the side trip are given from the end of West River Trail.

From the intersection of West River Trail with the trail that leads to Sawteeth and Gothics Mountains and Rainbow Falls, proceed east across the long bridge. On the other side of Ausable River, you intersect East River Trail to your left and a path to your right that heads uphill to Lake Road, as well as the trail to Indian Head and Fish Hawk Cliffs. Mileage given is from this point and does not include the total loop or the side trip to the cliffs.

Indian Head and Fish Hawk Cliffs

As you head uphill, you pass a maintenance building on your left and, shortly after, reach Lake Road. The road continues downhill to your right to where Adirondack Mountain Reserve (AMR) members have access to the Ausable Lakes. Hikers are prohibited from entering this area, so be mindful and keep on the designated trails. Head a short distance east along the road, and look for the trailhead on your right. The trail is marked with yellow disks, and you quickly reach what appears to be a fork in the trail. However, the trail on the right leads to an AMR boathouse and is private, so keep left. The trail has several switchbacks that make the ascent a little more enjoyable than

Ausable River: East River Trail

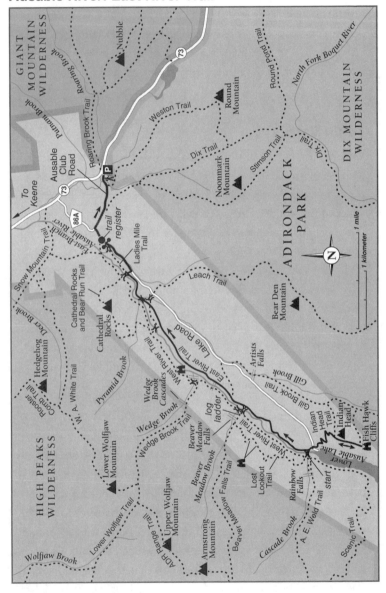

the typical rocky and straight scrambles to the top found on most Adirondacks trails. However, the trail is still considered steep, and several ladders have been built where short vertical sections over mossy and slick ledges would otherwise be difficult.

Approximately 0.3 mile in, you reach a fork in the trail and a sign indicating GOTHICS WINDOW—117 FEET to your right. The "window" is a slightly obscured view through the trees to the exposed portions of the Gothics. Though it's interesting, saplings threaten to engulf the view, and more-impressive vistas are found farther along the trail. The side trip doesn't take long, though, so you will probably find it worth the diversion.

You reach the first of the ladders shortly after this fork, and the zigzags become tight and more frequent. After climbing several ladders and switchbacks, the trail levels off briefly under the base of a mossy cliff that adds a neat feature along the trail. Views of the Gothics are more prominent now, and the trail, though steep, has fewer turns in it.

At 0.8 mile, you reach the crest of the ridge and a four-way intersection. To the left is Gill Brook Trail, straight ahead and down leads to Fish Hawk Cliffs, and to the right is the trail to Indian Head.

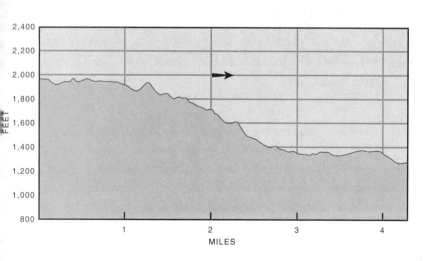

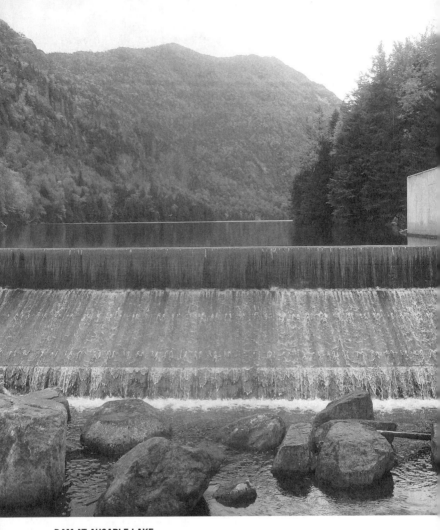

DAM AT AUSABLE LAKE

Thick evergreens now encompass the trail, and you briefly traverse the spine of this ridge before coming out on the exposed portions of the cliff that make up Indian Head. Spectacular views open up all around you, and you will quickly snap a dozen pictures. Rugged peaks with sheer cliffs fill the panorama to the north and west, but the most stunning views are of Lower Ausable Lake cradled between Colvin and Sawteeth Mountains. Continue along the exposed portion of bedrock along worn footpaths to a second, lower tier for a slightly different vantage point of the same spectacular view.

To reach Fish Hawk Cliffs, go back to the four-way intersection, and head down the trail, which is now on your right. The descent is steep and takes you down 160 feet into a col (saddle) near a pool called Wizard's Washbowl. Shortly ahead, 0.3 mile from the four-way intersection, you reach the cliffs, from which you have the interesting perspective of looking back upon Indian Head. To return, go back to the four-way intersection and straight down to Lake Road and then East River Trail.

East River Trail

East River Trail has fewer waterfalls than the west one but has its own unique character and elements that make it a great return trip. The trail meanders along the river briefly and then diverges east into the surrounding woods. Approximately 0.3 mile from the bridge, you navigate through a jumble of boulders that lie at the base of a cliff on your right. Shortly after, you pass Bullock Dam on your left. After the dam, the river levels off and flows through a grassy meadow. On the opposite shore, you see exposed cliffs and many views of the mountains to the west.

Just shy of a mile, you reach a fork in the trail; Beaver Meadow and the Gothics are to your left over a bridge and marked in blue, while East River Trail and the road, marked in red, continue straight ahead. Almost immediately after this intersection, you reach yet another fork, with East River Trail continuing straight ahead, and the road to your right.

The trail delves into tall and thick hemlocks, and you soon reach a beautiful waterfall along the river. You might remember seeing this more-than-20-foot-high waterfall and its constricted flume from the opposite shore. However, on this shore there are far better points from which to view the falls and its washed-out spillway. You are now high above the river canyon, and this is one of the last places to view the river. Farther on, you hear the rumble of the turbulent waters but will only have glimpses of the river from afar, as the trail winds its way back down to the gatehouse.

The trail becomes steep in a few sections but levels off about 2.5 miles from the start. Gill Brook joins you on your right, and shortly after this you will cross the brook over a bridge built from two sturdy beams. Soon after the bridge, you rejoin Ausable River as it flows northeast, and the trail follows the river 0.3 mile. At 3.1 miles, you reach another fork. Straight ahead is a bridge to West River Trail, while to your right is East River Trail and the path back to the road. In 0.1 mile, you will come in sight of the road. Follow it back to the gatehouse to sign out and then back to the parking area by NY 73, completing a trip of 4.3 miles from the bridge at Lower Ausable Lake, 10 miles to complete the loop, and a total of 11.6 miles, including the side trip.

Directions

The East River Trail begins at the end of the West River Trail, so the parking area is the same.

From I-87, take Exit 30 for US 9, and head north. Go 2.2 miles on US 9, and make a slight left onto NY 73. In 5.4 miles look for Ausable Club Road on your left just after descending a steep hill.

From the intersection of NY 9N and NY 73, head southeast on NY 73. In 6.1 miles, Ausable Club Road is on your right, directly across from the Giant Mountain parking area, described on page 276. The parking area is almost immediately on your left after you turn onto Ausable Club Road.

Giant's Nubble

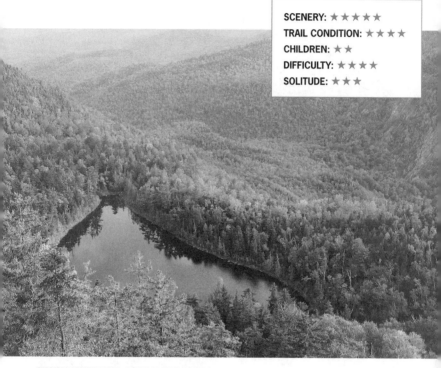

GIANT'S WASHBOWL SEEN ALONG DESCENT

SCENERY: ★ ★ ★ ★ ★
TRAIL CONDITION: ★ ★ ★ ★
CHILDREN: ★ ★
DIFFICULTY: ★ ★ ★ ★
SOLITUDE: ★ ★ ★

GPS COORDINATES: N44° 09.026'   W73° 46.027'

DISTANCE & CONFIGURATION: 4.4-mile loop

HIKING TIME: 3–4 hours

HIGHLIGHTS: Spectacular waterfall, primitive campsites, outstanding views

ELEVATION: 1,307' at trailhead, 2,750' at highest point

ACCESS: Open 24/7; no fees or permits required

MAPS: Giant Mountain Wilderness map: tinyurl.com/giantwildernessmap; National Geographic *Adirondack Park, Lake Placid/High Peaks* (#742)

FACILITIES: None

WHEELCHAIR ACCESS: No

CONTACTS: Giant Mountain Wilderness: www.dec.ny.gov/lands/100750.html; emergency contact: 518-891-0235

Giant's Nubble

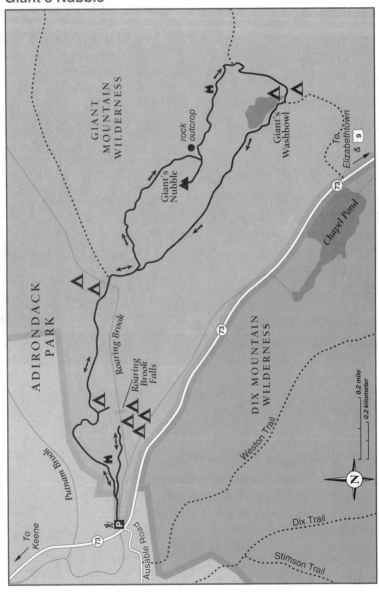

Overview

This trip combines a tall waterfall, scenic outlook, and picturesque pond within a very short distance. Don't let the distance or description fool you though; the rugged trail provides you with plenty of climbing, along with the majestic scenery associated with the High Peaks region.

Route Details

The asphalt parking area is tucked away on your right as you come down a steep hill along NY 73, so watch the odometer and be ready to make a sharp right. The parking area can easily accommodate a dozen cars, but if it's full, there is room on the shoulder of NY 73 or across the road in the Ausable River parking area (see its description on page 261).

The register and trailhead are at the eastern end of the lot.

The trail is broad and flat, and you can just barely glimpse Roaring Brook through hardwoods off to the right. During the peak of summer, the brook runs dry and indicates that the falls ahead may not be as majestic as during rainy conditions or during the winter melt. About 0.1 mile in, you reach a fork in the trail. To the right is the trail to the

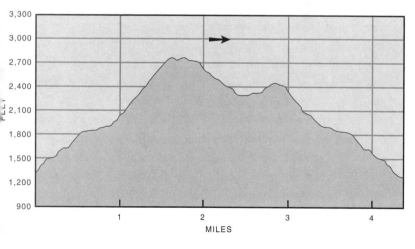

base of Roaring Brook Falls, while to the left the trail climbs to the top of the falls, Giant's Nubble, Giant's Washbowl, and Giant Mountain.

The Base of Roaring Brook Falls

Continue to the right past the sheer rock wall on your left until you reach Roaring Brook. Straight across the brook are four designated campsites. These sprawling sites lie under a thick canopy of tall hemlocks, and each has a large stone fire pit. They are shielded from view of the falls by a steep hill to the north but are fairly close to another stream, the outflow of Chapel Pond. The sound of the stream and the thundering of the falls will likely drown out the sound of the road, which is still close by, though the occasional loud vehicle might disturb the tranquil setting. To reach the falls, you have to scramble up the rocky brook a very short distance. The falls, the entirety of which can be seen from the road, are nearly 325 feet high, depending on where you measure the start. They cascade in three tiers, with only the lowest section visible at the base.

Giant's Nubble, Giant's Washbowl, and Giant Mountain

The trail climbs steadily from the fork and passes a tiny lookout shortly after you begin the ascent. After the first section of climbing, the trail levels off briefly and then climbs gently again as it winds briefly south around the contours of the hillside. As the trail swings east again, views across the valley begin to sprawl out before you. Approximately 0.5 mile in, you reach a fork in the trail; to your right are a designated campsite and the top of the falls, while straight ahead are Giant's Nubble, Giant's Washbowl, and the summit. The campsite, situated to the left of the falls path, is spacious, and there are plenty of spots to set up camp under the maple-and-ash canopy.

To reach the top of the falls, follow any of the footpaths to Roaring Brook, and then rock-hop downstream. From the top of the falls, very little of the waterfall is visible because the drop is so precipitous and the water flows through a deep cleft in the bedrock. However, there are spectacular views out to the western horizon. The rocks at the top of the falls have been worn smooth by innumerable visitors and slope gradually toward a sheer drop-off, so use extra caution, especially during wet conditions.

The main trail, marked by red disks, continues to head east and climbs steadily for the next 0.5 mile, where you reach another fork. To the left are two more designated campsites, both of which are situated under a heavy canopy of hemlocks and offer lots of room to set up. Shortly after this intersection, you wind around a large boulder and then turn quickly south as you rock-hop across Roaring Brook. On the opposite bank, you reach yet another fork. The trail to your left leads to the Giant Mountain summit, 2.5 miles, while the nubble and washbowl are off to your right. Trail signs indicate that the nubble and washbowl are both 0.9 mile away, but the actual mileage is roughly 0.3 mile less. A tenth of a mile ahead, you reach the fork where the trails to the nubble and washbowl diverge from each other. This is also the terminus of the loop around both features and a return point back to NY 73. A trail sign indicates that the nubble is still 0.9 mile ahead while the washbowl is 0.8 mile ahead on the right. You can hike the loop in either direction, though I recommend hiking the nubble first, as there are some truly stunning views of the washbowl as you descend.

The trail up to the nubble, now marked with yellow trail disks, is a bit rougher than sections previously covered but no more than the usual Adirondack trail.

Looming off to your left is the southern-exposed face of Giant Mountain, which can be glimpsed occasionally through the surrounding fir trees. Many portions of the trail traverse moss-covered bedrock, and you pass by a square ledge of this oddly lush rock on your right shortly before you reach the fork in the trail, at 1.6 miles, that leads to the nubble. Veering right at the fork, you quickly reach the southeastern tip of the nubble, and a vast panorama of the eastern High Peaks opens up before you. Footpaths weave in and out of the exposed, lichen-covered bedrock and wind-stunted fir trees as you make your way to the northern tip of the nubble. The lookout

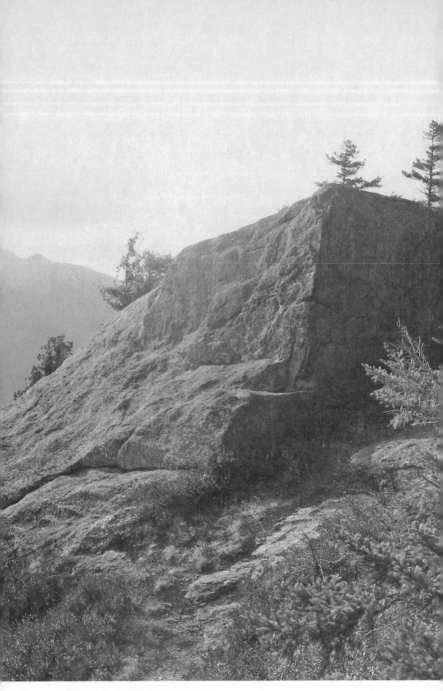

EXPOSED BEDROCK AT THE NUBBLE

reveals a panorama of the northern High Peaks, as well as a beautiful vista of Giant Mountain off to the east. If the drive into the region did not give you an appreciation of the ruggedness of this area, then the views from atop the nubble certainly will.

The descent to the washbowl, initially marked with yellow disks, can be quite steep but has numerous lookouts as well. Less than 0.3 mile from the nubble is a truly wonderful lookout that sits almost directly above the washbowl. The almost jet-black basin is nestled in a long depression between the base of the nubble and a ridgeline before the slope of the mountain precipitously drops more than 800 feet to the valley floor in less than 0.3 mile. From this vantage point, the pond seems to simply hang in the air. The trail weaves its way down through evergreens to the intersection with Giant's Ridge Trail at 2.1 miles. A green-and-white trail sign marks the intersection and indicates that the washbowl is a mere 0.3 mile farther on your right. The trail is heavily trodden but well maintained, and you quickly pass another designated campsite on your left, shortly before reaching the southeastern tip of the washbowl.

A path along the eastern shore of the pond leads to another designated campsite that sits close to the water's edge, but the main trail winds to your left. You quickly pass the last intersection along this loop, where trail signs indicate that the Chapel Pond parking area along NY 73 is 0.7 mile ahead on your left, marked in blue, while the trail back to Roaring Brook Falls continues to your right, with red markers. The rocky nubble looms over the washbowl and provides some dramatic scenery as you hike along the western ridge that contains the pond. The brief shoreline hike north is basically flat and rocky, with numerous rocks jutting out on the pond, all of which provide points from which to view the pond and nubble. After leaving the washbowl's shore, you climb briefly along the base of the nubble and then begin your descent back to the beginning of the nubble and washbowl loop.

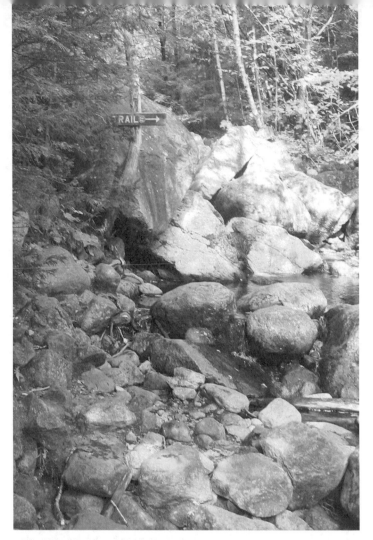

TRAIL CROSSING OF ROARING BROOK

Directions

From I-87, take Exit 30 for US 9, and head north. Go 2.2 miles on US 9, and make a slight left onto NY 73. In 5.4 miles the parking area is on your right, just after descending a steep hill; it's directly across from the southern intersection of Ausable Club Road and NY 73.

From the intersection of NY 9N and NY 73, head southeast on NY 73. In 6.1 miles, the parking area is on your left.

40

Hanging Spear Falls and Opalescent River

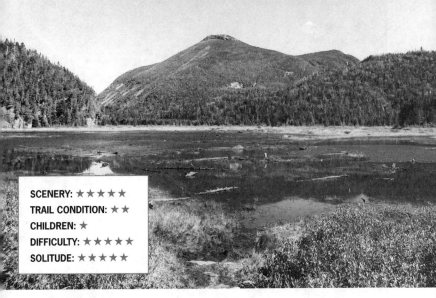

SCENERY: ★ ★ ★ ★ ★
TRAIL CONDITION: ★ ★
CHILDREN: ★
DIFFICULTY: ★ ★ ★ ★ ★
SOLITUDE: ★ ★ ★ ★

FLOWED LANDS

GPS COORDINATES: N44° 05.353'   W74° 03.381'

DISTANCE & CONFIGURATION: 13.7-mile loop or 11.0-mile out-and-back

HIKING TIME: 7.5–8.5 hours (overnight)

HIGHLIGHTS: Waterfall, remote lake, dramatic views

ELEVATION: 1,748' at trailhead, 2,800' at highest point

ACCESS: Open 24/7; no fees or permits required

MAPS: National Geographic *Adirondack Park, Lake Placid/High Peaks* (#742)

FACILITIES: Pit toilet at trailhead

WHEELCHAIR ACCESS: No

COMMENTS: While returning along East River Trail, there is a point where you will have to ford the Opalescent River, which could be hazardous during high water and/or cold weather. Water depth is commonly knee- or thigh-deep but is ankle-deep in summer/low water. No matter what, your feet will get wet, so plan accordingly.

CONTACTS: High Peaks Adirondack trail information: www.dec.ny.gov/outdoor/9198.html; emergency contact: 518-891-0235

Hanging Spear Falls and Opalescent River

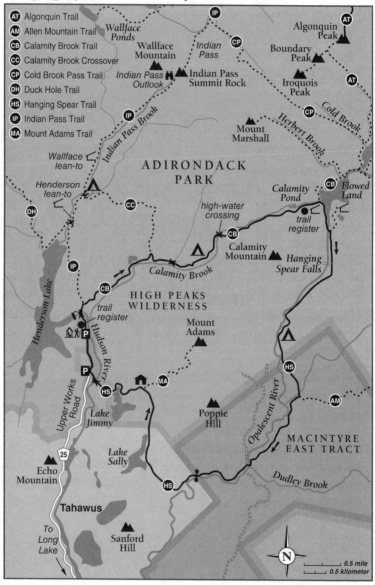

AT Algonquin Trail
AM Allen Mountain Trail
CB Calamity Brook Trail
CC Calamity Brook Crossover
CP Cold Brook Pass Trail
DH Duck Hole Trail
HS Hanging Spear Trail
IP Indian Pass Trail
MA Mount Adams Trail

Wallface
Ponds

Wallface
Mountain

Indian
Pass

Algonquin
Peak

Boundary
Peak

Indian Pass
Outlook

Indian Pass
Summit Rock

Iroquois
Peak

Cold Brook

Indian Pass Brook

Mount
Marshall

Herbert Brook

ADIRONDACK
PARK

Wallface
lean-to

Henderson
lean-to

Calamity
Pond

Flowed
Land

high-water
crossing

trail
register

Calamity
Mountain

Hanging
Spear Falls

Calamity Brook

HIGH PEAKS
WILDERNESS

Henderson Lake

trail
register

Hudson River

Mount
Adams

Upper Works
Road

Lake
Jimmy

Poppie
Hill

Opalescent River

MACINTYRE
EAST TRACT

Echo
Mountain

25

Lake
Sally

Dudley Brook

Tahawus

To
Long
Lake

Sanford
Hill

N

0.5 mile

0.5 kilometer

Overview

Deep in the remote High Peaks Wilderness is a stunning waterfall. Combine that with evocative names such as Hanging Spear, Flowed Lands, and Opalescent River and this adventure promises to be a spectacular trip, and it does not let you down. Because most hikers in the High Peaks are set on bagging the various peaks, chances are that you will be able to enjoy this isolated waterfall all to yourself. A protracted climb, a river ford, the remote location, and the length of the trail mean that this trip is best left to experienced hikers. You will want to give yourself plenty of time not only to complete the hike but also to enjoy the magnificent views at the falls and elsewhere along the loop.

Route Details

Note: Though the trip to the falls can be shortened to an 11.0-mile out-and-back by returning along the Calamity Brook Trail, completing the loop along the Hanging Spear Trail adds 2.6 miles but is not as rough and generally easier going—that is, the path is free of cobbles and requires less climbing. During winter or times of high water along the Opalescent River, the out-and-back route may be the only safe option. The full loop requires a full day and an early start, but

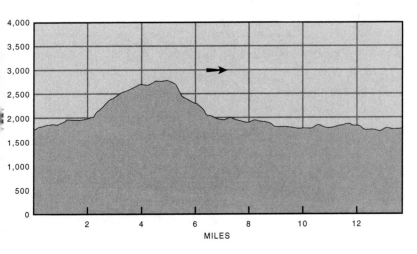

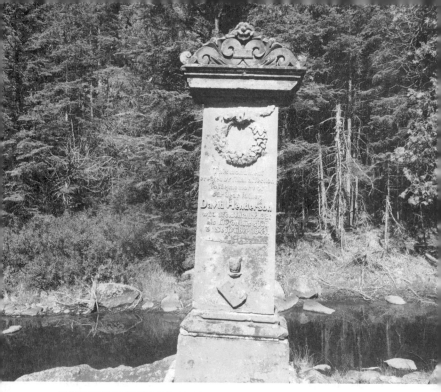

MONUMENT TO DAVID HENDERSON

the trail can also be treated as an overnight by either following the camping at-large rules laid out by the Department of Environmental Conservation (DEC) or by using designated camping areas and lean-tos mentioned within the description. The lean-tos at the end of the Calamity Brook Trail and within the Flowed Lands, four of which are readily accessible along the described route, are ideal spots to spend the night. There is also a designated campsite on the ascent, and a couple are located on the descent before reaching the Opalescent River crossing.

The Upper Works parking area is quite large and easily accommodates dozens of vehicles. The trail, marked with yellow disks, begins to the right of the trail register in the northeast corner of the lot. At roughly 0.25 mile you reach a wooden bridge that crosses the Hudson River. Just after the bridge, the road forks, with the trail continuing to the right. Just under 0.4 mile, you enter a meadow with a fork in the trail. The trail to the left leads to Duck Hole and Indian Pass (see page 289), marked with yellow disks, while the trail to the right is the Calamity Brook Trail, indicated here as Lake Colden Dam, Mount Marcy.

Continue along the right fork (east) following the red trail disks. The next mile of trail follows an old abandoned gravel road that weaves its way through rocks and boulders mostly out in the open. You will hear Calamity Brook shortly before the trail reaches it, a point where the brook makes a sharp southerly turn. The trail proceeds along an elevated berm between the tannin-colored Calamity Brook, with its bleached gravel banks on the right and a sprawling wetland on the left. From here forward, the trail more closely resembles the wooded foot trails that hikers are accustomed to.

A little over 0.3 mile ahead, 1.6 miles overall (despite what the trail sign reads), is another trail intersection. Straight and north, marked in red, is another route to Duck Hole and Indian Pass. To the right and over a bridge, marked in blue, is the continuation of the route to Mount Marcy via Lake Colden. Turn right and cross the tributary stream of Calamity Brook. The trail continues along level ground interspersed with a few mucky areas and soon rejoins Calamity Brook as the trail swings west. Shortly after passing a closed trail with a washed-out bridge on the right, you reach a tributary brook that you rock-hop across, after which the climbing to the Flowed Lands truly begins—roughly 800 feet gain over the next 2.5 miles.

Calamity Brook is no longer tannin laden and meandering but rather a crystal-clear babbling brook that tumbles through a boulder-strewn bed. The trail weaves its way to and from the brook as you ascend. You pass a camping disk on the right at 2.7 miles, about midway up a hill, before the trail levels out briefly at a wet area. This is one of many long mires that trail crews have tried to bypass with logs, log-and-plank boardwalks, and other configurations that vary in success in keeping your boots dry and keeping you out of the muck. At some point along the climb, you will likely have to trudge through the muck, but not here.

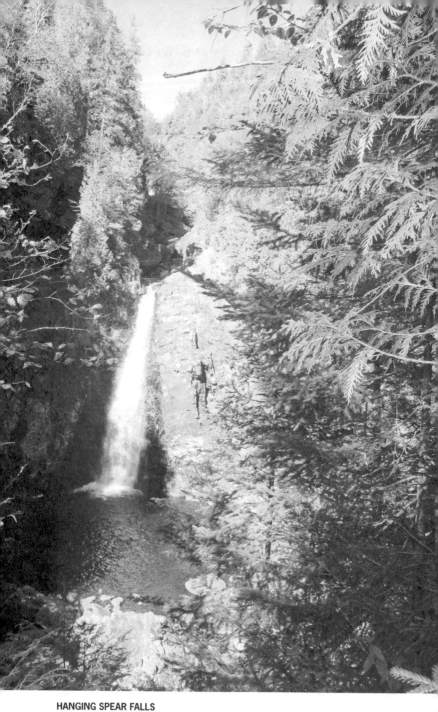

HANGING SPEAR FALLS

At roughly 3 miles reach an unmarked fork in the trail just before reintersecting Calamity Brook. During most of the year, you can cross Calamity Brook by rock-hopping, but during times of high water and flooding, mostly during the spring, you will want to continue uphill and to the left to the high-water crossing: a cable bridge that was replaced after floodwaters from Hurricane Irene washed out the previous bridge in 2011. The high-water bypass reconnects with the main trail a little uphill on the opposite bank.

The trail continues to climb steadily past this crossing, and you will encounter a series of wet and mucky areas that become increasingly harder to navigate. Calamity Brook flows down to your left, and much of the trail resembles a cobble-strewn brook in its own right. As the trail nears the top of the climb, it emerges from the surrounding forest into an open upland wetland, roughly 4 miles from the start. The trail swings around the southern and eastern edges of the wetland that surrounds Calamity Pond. A short side path found along the southern edge takes you through the encircling shrubs and provides a photo opportunity of the upland wetland. As you near the northeastern edge of the wetland, keep an eye out for a worn footpath leading north, located just before the trail bends east and away from the wetland. This short trail will take you to the headwaters of the pond and a stone monument dedicated to David Henderson, who died from an accidental gunshot here in 1845. You'll find another scenic view of the wetland and pond at the inlet.

Back along the main trail, continue east, through one long boot-sucking mire, and soon reach the Calamity #1 Lean-To and trail register for the inner High Peaks Wilderness. (There are special regulations for the inner High Peaks, mostly regarding camping and the use of bear-resistant canisters. For camping rules, see www.dec .ny.gov/outdoor/7872.html; for information on bear-resistant canisters, see www.dec.ny.gov/animals/7225.html.) A major trail intersection is also located at the trail register. To the left and marked in red are the trails leading to Lake Colden Dam, Avalanche Lake, and Mount Marcy. Straight ahead and marked in red are the trails to Flowed Lands and Hanging Spear Falls. Continue straight (east) and quickly reach a short path leading down to the eastern edge of the Flowed Lands, where a sprawling panorama of a winding wetland is framed by Mount Colden to the east and the foot of Mount Marshall to the west. It's a stunning scene and a good spot to break, as the next best stop, the Flowed Lands Lean-To a little farther on, is likely occupied. Alternatively, wait until you reach the lookout opposite Hanging Spear Falls, a truly amazing and tranquil setting, 1 mile farther.

Heading south and away from this vista, the trail heads uphill briefly before descending into a depression just in front of the Flowed Lands Lean-To, 4.7 miles. At this point it is not immediately apparent where the trail continues. With the lean-to straight ahead, look right and scramble uphill, where you find red trail disks and a sign leading to a nearby pit toilet and the trail becomes more evident. Continue heading nearly due south another 0.3 mile to where you reach the end of the Flowed Lands and the head of the Opalescent River.

You will hear the sounds of the outflow of the Flowed Lands a short distance before you reach the crossing point just upstream from the old dam. The dam was originally created by the McIntyre Iron Works, which the aforementioned David Henderson helped establish, but the dam was deemed unsafe and was breached by the DEC in 1984. Scramble down from the trail to the gravel beach. Red trail disks are visible on the opposite shore, and you will have to pick your way atop a collection of rocks that loosely form a bridge across.

Once atop the opposite bank, you reach a trail intersection; to the left and marked in yellow is the Livingstone Point Lean-To, 0.4 mile away, while the path forward is to the right (south) following red trail disks. As you begin heading south along East River Trail, look immediately to the right for a point where you can snap a few pictures atop an old section of the dam. Nearby, a sign warns that the bridge across the Opalescent River, 4.2 miles farther along the trail, is out and you will have to ford the river. As the sign indicates, this could be hazardous during high water and during cold weather because inevitably you will have to wade or at the minimum get your feet wet during the crossing.

As the trail leads south to Hanging Spear Falls, it follows the Opalescent River quite closely along a narrow footpath. Long strands of algae cling to river rock, giving the river a green tinge. And though you may think that the green algae is the source of the river's name, the name was given by a state geologist who found the riverbed filled with opalescent feldspar, also known as labradorite. Under the right conditions the labradorite looks blue, and sometimes green, bronze, gold, or even iridescent. About 0.25 mile along the descent, a small unnamed waterfall, really a flume, with a small pool can be found among car-sized boulders. Farther along the trail you will hear other small waterfalls just out of sight, and you may be tempted to bushwhack in to see if they are Hanging Spear Falls, but rest assured, the site to view the actual falls is evident. Indeed a sign with an arrow indicates that the "falls" are available along a side trail, a little less than 0.5 mile from the crossing, 5.5 miles overall.

Once on the side trail, follow it a short way to the viewing area, a flat spot directly south of the falls. It might be tempting to try to descend a worn herd path visible to the side of the trail, but this path is dangerous, easily eroded, and likely to get you injured, if not trapped, near the base of the falls. At the viewing area, the surrounding canopy perfectly frames the 75-foot-high falls, and there is even an ideally placed root upon which you can sit and admire the majestic view. If you look upstream you will see not only Hanging Spear Falls but also a series of falls farther north. Incidentally, the falls are so named because during full flow they tend to bifurcate and give the appearance of a spearhead suspended in the air. This is only during times of high flow, but even at modest flow the falls are impressive.

To continue along the trail, you can either backtrack to the main trail or continue along the side trail, which loops back to the main trail a little farther downhill. Continue downhill on the main trail, and soon reach a brook crossing, the first along this section of trail and a useful landmark in case you missed the lookout side trail. For the next

0.75 mile the trail winds its way through dense understory out of ear-shot and sight of the river. Shortly after the Opalescent River comes back into view, some 40–50 feet below, the trail winds down to a point directly along its banks. The trail then weaves along the eastern bank through some mucky sections and then crosses a gravel outwash of the river high water/old riverbed near a designated campsite 0.3 mile ahead, 6.8 miles overall. This marks the end of the descent, and the rest of the trail follows mostly level ground.

Gradually the trail leads away from the river and climbs slightly to a clearing among a network of old access/logging roads. An arrow staked in the clearing indicates that the trail follows the western edge of this clearing. At 7.6 miles reach Upper Twin Brook, which is eas-ily crossed atop several large boulders just downstream on the right. On the other side, pass an informal campsite and soon reach a trail intersection. Left is the trail to Allen Mountain, while right, follow-ing yellow trail markers, is the continuation of East River Trail to the Upper Works trailhead parking.

The trail now follows a narrow, worn path that heads gen-erally southwest through open fields dotted with small evergreens and raspberry bushes. Hiking in the open is indeed a change of scenery from the typical forested trails and provides some interest-ing views of Calamity Mountain and Mount Adams to the north and west, while Allen Mountain looms to the east; you will have to turn around to catch this photo op. For the next 1.2 miles this setting is dominant with only a few exceptions; the most notable is 0.25 mile ahead, where the trail delves briefly into the forest and crosses Lower Twin Brook.

At roughly 9 miles, after reentering the forest, the trail leads down to the banks over the Opalescent River once again. Bear left and follow the river another 0.1 mile to where it broadens at the designated crossing. Dozens of feet across at low water, the cross-ing necessitates getting your feet wet and/or wading, depending on the depth. Once across, turn left and follow an old road south; no trail markers are readily apparent, but the wide access road is easy to

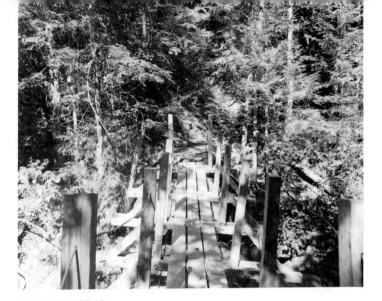

HIGH-WATER BRIDGE

follow. The Opalescent is now broad and meandering as it accompanies you on the left as the trail gradually swings east.

A little over 0.75 mile from the crossing, 9.9 miles overall, reach a red vehicle-barrier gate close to a point where the Opalescent turns sharply south. Past the barrier gate, the road continues southwest awhile but gradually begins to curve northwest. Sanford Hill can be seen off to the left, while Popple Hill dominates the view to the right. A half mile past the barrier gate and at a point heading nearly due north, the trail departs from the road and continues along a worn footpath. Rocks and branches are laid across the road, and you will see a yellow trail arrow on the right through the foliage.

The trail follows an almost due-north course, and within 0.3 mile you can glimpse Lake Sally through the surrounding forest on the left. This is the southern bay of Lake Sally, and after briefly diverting into the surrounding forest about 0.25 mile, you reach its northern bay. The trail climbs slightly around this bay and intersects a slightly overgrown gravel road, roughly 11.2 miles overall. Bear right and follow this road another 0.3 mile north to where it bends left (northwest) near where an old logging road continues straight ahead. A quarter mile farther, and roughly 0.6 mile from the intersection with the road, pass the trail to Mount Adams, marked in red on the right. Just a little farther, reach two green buildings, the Mount Adams fire tower cabins.

The trail bears left (south) at the cabins and soon bends west and quickly reaches the northern bay of Lake Jimmy, less than 0.3 mile from the cabins, 12.3 miles overall. Old maps show a bridge crossing this bay, but the bridge no longer connects the two shores; beaver activity had undermined it to the point that it was no longer safe. To get around the bay, turn right and head north, where logs and planks help you navigate through the wetland that surrounds Lake Jimmy. Soon the trail swings west and you cross the two outlets of Jimmy in quick succession. After turning left and briefly heading south, reconnect with the old trail, and head due west through a deep forest another 0.25 mile to where you intersect the Hudson River once again. A suspended steel-grate bridge with fenced-in sides carries you high above the Hudson. Once on the other side, it is a short distance to the East River Trail parking area. Turn right onto Upper Works Road, and continue 0.75 mile to the Upper Works trailhead and parking area for a round-trip of 13.7 miles.

Directions

FROM THE WEST   From the intersection of NY 30 and NY 28N in Long Lake, head 18.9 miles east along NY 28N, and turn left onto Blue Ridge Road. At 0.3 mile Tahawus Road/County Road 25 merges with Blue Ridge Road on the left. Continue 0.9 mile, 1.2 miles from NY 28N, and bear left onto Tahawus Road/CR 25. After another 6.3 miles bear left onto Upper Works Road/CR 25A. Continue north another 3.5 miles to the end of the road and the Upper Works parking area.

FROM ALL OTHER POINTS   From I-87 take Exit 29 toward Newcomb/North Hudson. Head 17.5 miles west along Blue Ridge Road/CR 84, and turn right onto Tahawus Road/CR 25. At 6.3 miles, bear left onto Upper Works Road/CR 25A. Continue north another 3.5 miles to the end of the road and the Upper Works parking area.

41

Indian Pass

SCENERY: ★ ★ ★ ★
TRAIL CONDITION: ★ ★ ★
CHILDREN: ★ ★ ★
DIFFICULTY: ★ ★ ★
SOLITUDE: ★ ★ ★ ★ ★

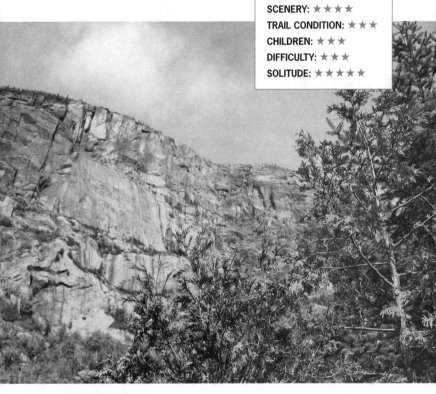

WALLFACE MOUNTAIN

GPS COORDINATES: N44° 05.353'   W74° 03.382'

DISTANCE & CONFIGURATION: 8.8-mile out-and-back

HIKING TIME: 5–6 hours

HIGHLIGHTS: Maze of boulders, sheer cliffs, panoramic views

ELEVATION: 1,758' at trailhead, 2,855' at highest point

ACCESS: Open 24/7; no fees or permits required

MAPS: National Geographic *Adirondack Park, Lake Placid/High Peaks* (#742)

FACILITIES: Pit toilet at the parking area

WHEELCHAIR ACCESS: No

CONTACTS: High Peaks Adirondack trail information: www.dec.ny.gov/outdoor/9198.html; emergency contact: 518-891-0235

Indian Pass

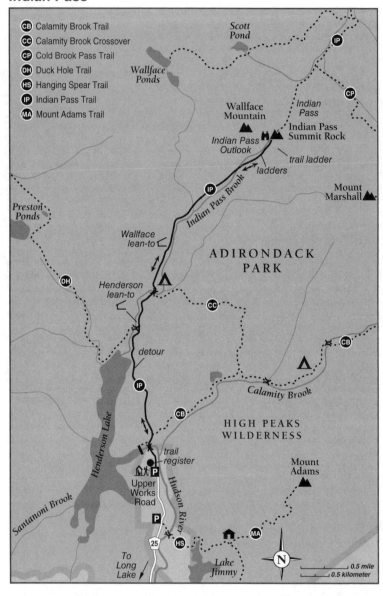

CB Calamity Brook Trail
CC Calamity Brook Crossover
CP Cold Brook Pass Trail
DH Duck Hole Trail
HS Hanging Spear Trail
IP Indian Pass Trail
MA Mount Adams Trail

Scott Pond

Wallface Ponds

Wallface Mountain

Indian Pass

Indian Pass Summit Rock

Indian Pass Outlook

trail ladder

ladders

Mount Marshall

Indian Pass Brook

Preston Ponds

ADIRONDACK PARK

Wallface lean-to

Henderson lean-to

Calamity Brook Crossover

detour

Calamity Brook

Henderson Lake

HIGH PEAKS WILDERNESS

trail register

Mount Adams

Upper Works Road

Santanoni Brook

Hudson River

25

To Long Lake

Lake Jimmy

N

0.5 mile
0.5 kilometer

Overview

The trail leading to Indian Pass is an enjoyable excursion in its own right, and you can't help but feel the remoteness of the High Peaks Wilderness that surrounds you. The first three-quarters of the trail is, however, not that different from many deep-woods hikes. It's the last 0.8 mile that really sets this trail apart and makes it a must-have adventure. After navigating your way through a maze of enormous boulders, you soon reach Summit Rock, and the spectacle of Wallface Mountain is truly impressive.

Route Details

The Upper Works parking area for Indian Pass is quite large and easily accommodates dozens of vehicles. Indeed, it is one of the major access points for the High Peaks Wilderness and all the adventure that the area encompasses. The trail, marked with yellow disks, begins to the right of the trail register in the northeast corner of the lot. The trail starts along a gravelly road within the boundaries of the Tahawus Preserve, a vast area of wilderness that was acquired by the Open Space Institute in 2003, with major sections now jointly managed by the institute and the Department of Environmental Conservation.

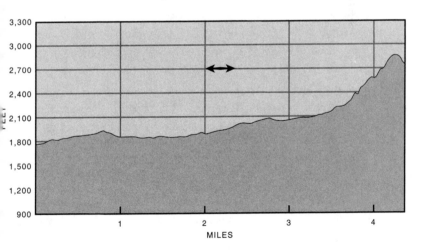

After 0.3 mile, you reach a wooden bridge sturdy enough for vehicles to cross. Congratulations! You have just crossed the Hudson River at its headwater. Just after the bridge, the road forks, with the trail continuing on the right. At 0.4 mile you enter a meadow with a fork in the trail. The trail to the left leads to Duck Hole and Indian Pass, marked with yellow disks, while the trail to the right, marked with red disks, is Calamity Brook Trail and Mount Marcy via Lake Colden. Calamity Brook Trail is also the return trip if you decide to take an extended trip, day or overnight, by crossing over the McIntyre Mountains via Cold Brook Pass.

Continue along the left trail, which is a mostly open road with occasional views of Lake Henderson on your left. The road has many muddy areas, and regrowth encroaches in several places. At 1.1 miles, you encounter what appears to be a fork but is actually a route around a mucky area. Choose the right-hand path to avoid the worst of the mud. Just after this rerouting, you come close to Lake Henderson again, but thick hemlocks obscure most of the view.

Indian Pass Brook now flows off to your left, and at 1.5 miles, you reach another fork in the trail. At this point, you leave the broad road and stick to the foot trails. To the left is a log-and-plank bridge, and signs indicate that the Duck Hole Lean-To is 5.3 miles and Coreys, 23.3 miles. Similarly, the sign indicates Henderson Lean-To is 0.2 mile, Indian Pass is 2.7 miles, and the Adirondak Loj is 10.4 miles straight ahead. (The mileage to the Loj must include a detour because a straight path along the entire Indian Pass Trail brings you to the Loj in 10.4 miles, and you have already hiked 1.5 miles.)

Continue straight along mostly flat terrain, now marked with red disks. In 1.7 miles you pass the Henderson Lean-To on your left. On a Saturday morning this lean-to is usually filled with hikers who started late on Friday and want to get moving early. After reaching a meadow Indian Pass Brook is again within sight, and you quickly reach the last fork of this trip, 2.1 miles. Signs indicate that to the left, Wallface Lean-To is 0.6 mile, Indian Pass is 2.3 miles, and the Adirondak Loj is 6 miles. (Once again, the mileage to the Loj seems

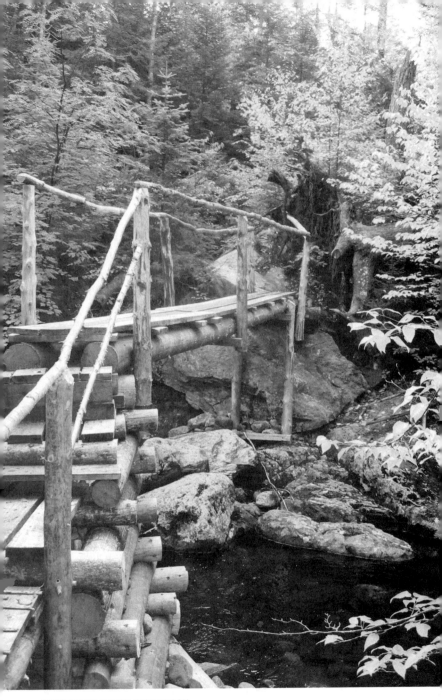

BRIDGE OVER INDIAN PASS BROOK

to be mistaken, but the others are correct.) The trail straight ahead, marked in blue, is the Calamity Brook Crossover trail, with Calamity Brook at 2.1 miles and Lake Colden at 6 miles.

After taking the left trail, marked in red, you quickly reach a bridge over Indian Pass Brook. The recently constructed bridge has round rails and posts, as well as a large, rock-filled crib on the opposite shore. Shortly after reaching the opposite shore, you pass a minor fork in the trail and a yellow disk indicating a designated campsite to your right. Nestled among dense evergreen saplings, the site is close to the confluence of two streams. The site has a sheltered feel and is filled with the soft babbling sounds of the water nearby.

Indian Pass Brook now flows on your right, and though it is nearby, you don't really see the brook until you approach the Wallface Lean-To, 2.7 miles. The trail passes within feet of the brook, and the lean-to is just to the left of the trail. This is perhaps an ideal spot to enjoy the brook, but if you plan to stay in the lean-to, then expect traffic. The trail is mostly flat, and you cross many seasonal feeder streams as you work your way northeast to the intersection of a seasonal stream and Indian Pass Brook. You cross and recross the stream in what is a muddy little delta extending about 0.1 mile. Past this mire, Indian Pass Brook continues to flow on your right. The grade steadily increases, and soon a sheer rock wall begins to rise on your right. At 3.8 miles a jumble of enormous boulders on the eastern shore invites exploration. This is fortunate, as the trail crosses over Indian Pass Brook at this point, but the markings for the crossing are not that clear, and it's easy to miss the exact crossover point.

On the other shore, the trail becomes more rugged and climbs steeply in sections. The moss-covered, giant boulders through which you are climbing form myriad crevices, caves, and clefts that make for interesting scenery and exploration. As you climb, and after passing a 40-foot-high boulder on your right, you will begin to glimpse through the canopy to your left the sheer rock walls of Wallface Mountain. The scene is impressive and promises a dramatic vista ahead at Indian Pass Outlook. At 4.1 miles you reach a series of short ladders that assist you up this steep section. The trail swings south briefly, then heads north again to the base of a much taller ladder at 4.3 miles. Once you are atop this ladder, it is a very short way to the fork that leads to the outlook on your left. A short ladder leads you a few dozen feet off the main trail to the Indian Pass Summit Rock outlook. From this rocky outcrop, you have an amazing view of the sheer cliffs of Wallface Mountain, as well as an expansive view down the valley to the south. Return the way you came for a total trip of 8.8 miles.

Directions

FROM THE WEST   From the intersection of NY 30 and NY 28N in Long Lake, head 18.9 miles east along NY 28N, and turn left onto Blue Ridge Road. At 0.3 mile Tahawus Road/County Road 25 merges with Blue Ridge Road on the left. Continue 0.9 mile, 1.2 miles from NY 28N, and bear left onto Tahawus/CR 25. After another 6.3 miles bear left onto Upper Works Road/CR 25A. Continue north another 3.5 miles to the end of the road and the Upper Works parking area.

FROM ALL OTHER POINTS   From I-87 take Exit 29 toward Newcomb/North Hudson. Head 17.5 miles west along Blue Ridge Road/CR 84, and turn right onto Tahawus Road/CR 25. At 6.3 miles bear left onto Upper Works Road/CR 25A. Continue north another 3.5 miles to the end of the road and the Upper Works parking area.

42

Algonquin Peak

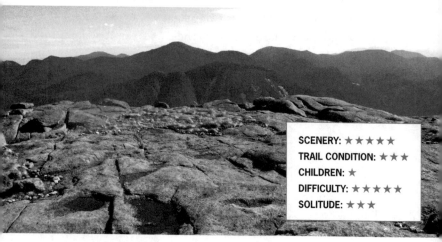

ATOP ALGONQUIN PEAK

GPS COORDINATES: N44° 10.969' W73° 57.746'

DISTANCE & CONFIGURATION: 8.0-mile out-and-back, 0.8-mile out-and-back side trip to Wright Peak

HIKING TIME: 7–8 hours

HIGHLIGHTS: Bald mountain(s), alpine ecosystems, panoramic views, waterfall

ELEVATION: 2,179' at trailhead, 5,115' at highest point

ACCESS: Open 24/7; $5 for Adirondack Mountain Club members, $10 per day for non-members. During summer and holiday weekends the lots fill quickly and are at capacity by early afternoon. When parking booth is closed, pay and register with the self-service box. Parking is free for guests staying at the Loj/Wilderness Campground.

MAPS: National Geographic *Adirondack Park, Lake Placid/High Peaks* (#742)

FACILITIES: Changing rooms, bathrooms, showers, information center

WHEELCHAIR ACCESS: No

COMMENTS: Be aware that Algonquin Peak (and Wright Peak if you choose the optional side trip) is an alpine zone. You won't find this ecosystem anywhere in New York except atop the highest of the High Peaks. While this makes for a great experience, the vegetation is also rare, fragile, and endangered. Stepping or sitting on these plants *will kill them* and destroy the habitat. As such, avoid any vegetation in these zones, and only walk along designated trails and solid rock surfaces.

CONTACTS: High Peaks trail information: www.dec.ny.gov/outdoor/9198.html; emergency contact: 518-891-0235

Overview

At 5,115 feet, Algonquin Peak is the second-highest peak in New York (Mount Marcy stands at 5,343 feet tall). Those starting or looking to complete their 46 High Peak challenge can easily add Wright Peak (side trip detailed on page 300) and Iroquois Mountain to their list. Not only are the views atop Algonquin and Wright Peaks stunning, but the alpine ecosystem is unique to all but a few places in New York. The ascent is nearly 3,000 feet to Algonquin alone, so plan on taking considerably more time along this trail than the 8-mile trek would normally suggest.

Note: If you want a little more adventure, add the return along Avalanche Pass (see page 304), extending the trip by nearly 4 miles and 2 hours.

Route Details

Parking at the Loj is extensive and could easily accommodate 100 (or more) cars in the various gravel parking lots. However, this is a major starting point for hikers and backpackers looking to explore the remote heart of the High Peaks wilderness, so the lot fills to capacity during the summer and holiday weekends. Many of the people exploring the region will be on extended overnight treks, and the lot provides access to a wide network of trails. But the trail network in the interior is so extensive that although you will pass by other hikers, it won't be as frequently as the number of cars seems to indicate.

The trailhead and register are found near a kiosk on the eastern edge of the parking area. The initial section of the trail, marked with blue disks, lies within the Adirondack Mountain Club's boundaries and has received extensive trail work/maintenance to accommodate the heavy traffic that passes through the area. At roughly 0.3 mile reach a long boardwalk that traverses a wetland along MacIntyre Brook. About 0.4 mile farther, reach the intersection with the Fangorn Forest Trail and the Department of Environmental Conservation High Peaks Wilderness boundary, 0.7 mile. Bear left and

Algonquin Peak

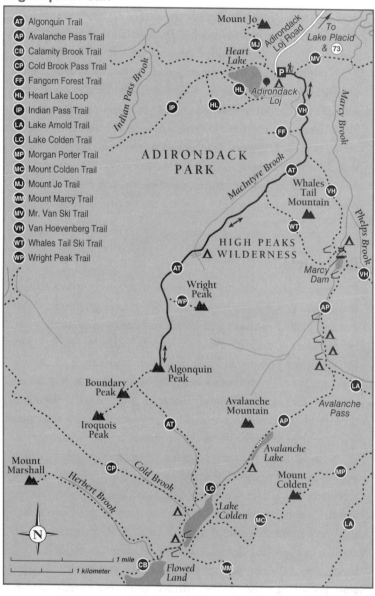

AT Algonquin Trail
AP Avalanche Pass Trail
CB Calamity Brook Trail
CP Cold Brook Pass Trail
FF Fangorn Forest Trail
HL Heart Lake Loop
IP Indian Pass Trail
LA Lake Arnold Trail
LC Lake Colden Trail
MP Morgan Porter Trail
MC Mount Colden Trail
MJ Mount Jo Trail
MM Mount Marcy Trail
MV Mr. Van Ski Trail
VH Van Hoevenberg Trail
WT Whales Tail Ski Trail
WP Wright Peak Trail

Mount Jo
Adirondack Loj Road
To Lake Placid & 73
Heart Lake
MJ
MV
P
HL
Adirondack Loj
HL
IP
VH
Indian Pass Brook
FF
ADIRONDACK PARK
MacIntyre Brook
AT
Marcy Brook
Whales Tail Mountain
VH
Phelps Brook
WT
HIGH PEAKS WILDERNESS
Marcy Dam
VH
AT
Wright Peak
WP
AP
Boundary Peak
Algonquin Peak
LA
Iroquois Peak
AT
Avalanche Mountain
AP
Avalanche Pass
Mount Marshall
CP
Cold Brook
Avalanche Lake
Herbert Brook
LC
Mount Colden
MP
Lake Colden
MC
LA
N
CB
Flowed Land
MM

1 mile
1 kilometer

continue following blue trail disks as the trail climbs gradually, with MacIntyre Brook flowing 20–30 feet below. At 1 mile reach the first major trail intersection. To the left, marked in blue, are the Marcy Dam lean-tos, Avalanche Lake, Lake Colden, and Mount Marcy; this is the return leg of the Avalanche Pass loop. Straight, marked in yellow, is Whales Tail, as well as Wright and Algonquin Peaks.

Continue straight (south) as you begin the steadily increasing ascent to Algonquin Peak—more than 2,800 feet over the next 3 miles. Just 0.5 mile farther, pass the intersection with the Whales Tail Trail on the left, just before crossing a seasonal brook that feeds MacIntyre Brook. There are several of these seasonal stream crossings along the initial portion of the ascent, with a notable one roughly 0.5 mile ahead, where a trail arrow indicates a crossing among several large boulders. The deciduous forest begins to give way to paper birches and firs as the climbing continues. Shortly after negotiating a very steep portion of bedrock that may require use of your hands, the sound of water beckons you on to what is the best spot to stop and take a break along the climb. Just before 2.6 miles—more than halfway in distance but less than half of the ascent (at only 1,200 of the 2,800 feet to be climbed)—is a stunning waterfall. The unnamed

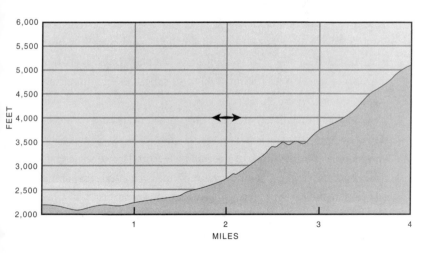

fall, which is the source of MacIntyre Brook, is roughly 30–40 feet high, with a modest flow and a shallow pool at its base.

Past the waterfall, the trail continues its steep ascent where dense saplings enclose the trail. At roughly 2.9 miles reach a pass between Wright Peak to the east and a sheer vertical cliff to the west. At this juncture signs warn about being prepared for ice and snow, which can come as early as October and as late as May. Do not take this warning lightly, as long sections of trail are along exposed bedrock, which when covered in ice are dangerous or impassable without proper equipment (crampons, ice ax, warm clothing). Additionally, snow is considerably deeper than in the parking area where you started. **Do not proceed** during the winter if you are not prepared. Every year severe injuries and fatalities occur when people ignore these warnings.

A little less than 0.5 mile more of scrambling and climbing, reach the intersection with the Wright Peak Trail on the left. The side trip, indicated with blue trail markers and described below, is highly recommended. But remember, more than 1,000 feet of climbing is required to reach Algonquin Peak from this point.

Side Trip to Wright Peak
(adds 0.8 mile and 600' of climbing)
For anyone wishing to work on their 46 High Peak bucket list, now is the time to bag one more: Wright Peak. The side trip is steep, but the view is worth it and hints at what to expect when summiting Algonquin farther on.

Almost immediately after starting the ascent, reach a wide section of bedrock that you will have to scramble up. In winter this slide may be a sheet of ice. Much of the trail is steep and traverses ledges, with short firs hugging tight to the trail until you reach the alpine zone. A sign indicates when you are entering this zone, just beneath a steep rock wall that you will have to climb. Once on top, the trees disappear, and you enter a stark and comparatively barren environment.

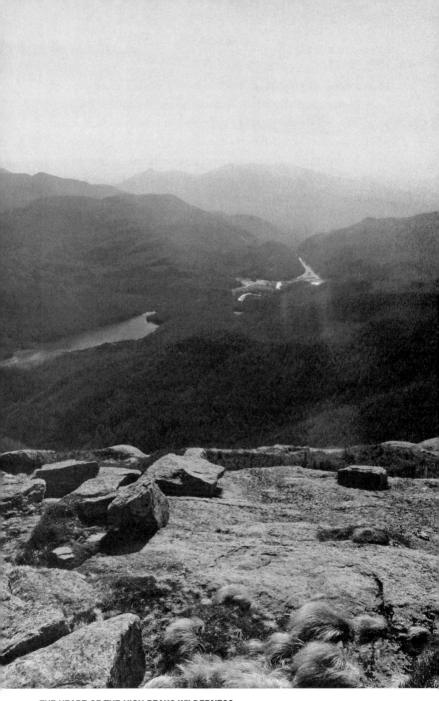

THE HEART OF THE HIGH PEAKS WILDERNESS

Lichens, clumps of grass, and wind-stunted evergreens precariously cling to what little nutrients they can get along the wind-scraped peak. You still have a ways to climb, but with the peak in sight you will happily push on up the steep slope.

Without trees for trail markers, you will have to rely on painted spots along ledges, rock cairns, and various pebble-lined paths. Remember, you do not want to step on any vegetation, so be mindful of where you traverse. Once atop, you will find a stunning 360-degree panorama of the High Peaks, including your next stop: Algonquin Peak, looming 500 feet above to the south. Return the way you came, again being careful where you traverse.

Back along the main trail continue south, follow yellow markers and continue the climb (more than 1,100 feet over the next roughly 0.6 mile) to Algonquin Peak. Within 0.25 mile, reach a very steep section of trail that ascends along an exposed portion of bedrock. To make your way up the sheer rock face, you will have to find foot- and handholds on small clefts and deformities in the rock. Complicating matters, water flows over the face and ice is likely when temperatures are below freezing. I found that the right side of the trail seemed to have more places for "steps" and handholds. After this protracted climb, the trail is more easily traversed, with large slabs of rock often forming steps along the climb.

About 0.25 mile past the sheer climb, reach the beginning of the alpine zone. Unlike Wright Peak, there is significantly more climbing to be done above the alpine zone boundary, and the peak is never quite in sight to lure you onward. To navigate through the alpine zone, remember to walk only on the designated path or exposed rock. To find the path, look for paint on the rocks, rock cairns for the direction of travel, and pebble walls that separate the trail from the vegetative areas. There is still roughly 0.25 mile and more than 300 feet of elevation to go until the actual summit. As you climb to the alpine zone, your whole perspective changes; the trees are gone and nothing remains but rock and low-lying vegetation clinging to scraps of soil caught in the cleft of rocks or in the lee of boulders. Often wind whips over the summit, making it hard to hear, but the barren landscape is stunning. The peak is broad and spread out, with a dramatic panorama of the High Peaks Wilderness Area all around you. Only Mount Marcy, about 3.8 miles southeast, is higher, and on clear days the horizon seems endless. While you look about the summit and take in the view, once again be careful of the fragile ecosystem.

If it took you longer than expected to reach the summit or if weather or night threatens, then you should seriously consider returning the way you came. But if time, weather, and energy are on your side, then I recommend the return leg along Avalanche Pass. The route heads deeper into the High Peaks Wilderness and will take considerably more time and effort to complete. But after a bone-jarring descent, you traverse some areas that, combined with the trip to Algonquin, make for one of the most scenic routes you could take in the Adirondacks. Should you choose that route, the total trip length (without the side trip to Wright) would be 11.8 miles; otherwise, return the way you came for a trip length of 8.0 miles.

Directions

From the intersection of NY 73 and NY 86 in Lake Placid, head 3.3 miles south on NY 73, and follow the directions below. From the intersection of NY 73 and NY 9N in downtown Keene, head 10.9 miles west on NY 73, and follow the directions below.

Turn south onto Adirondack Loj Road. Continue 5.1 miles to the vehicle-entry booth, and the main parking area is on the left past the visitor center.

43 # Avalanche Pass

SCENERY: ★ ★ ★ ★ ★
TRAIL CONDITION: ★
CHILDREN: ★
DIFFICULTY: ★ ★ ★ ★ ★
SOLITUDE: ★ ★ ★ ★

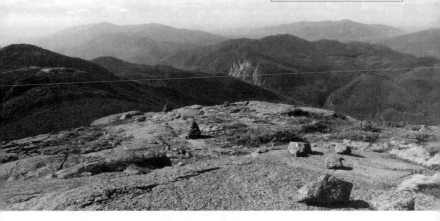

THE SOUTHERN SLOPE OF ALGONQUIN PEAK

GPS COORDINATES: Loj parking area: N44° 10.969' W73° 57.746'
Algonquin Peak: N44° 8.611' W73° 59.223'

DISTANCE & CONFIGURATION: 11.8-mile loop (includes the Algonquin Peak trail, page 296)

HIKING TIME: 8.5–9.5 hours

HIGHLIGHTS: Remote lake, dramatic cliffs, panoramic views, waterfalls

ELEVATION: 5,115' at Algonquin summit; 2,091' at lowest point

ACCESS: Open 24/7; $5 for Adirondack Mountain Club members, $10 per day for non-members. During summer and holiday weekends the lots fill quickly and are at capacity by early afternoon. When parking booth is closed, pay and register with the self-service box. Parking is free for guests staying at the Loj/Wilderness Campground.

MAPS: National Geographic *Adirondack Park, Lake Placid/High Peaks* (#742)

FACILITIES: Changing rooms, bathrooms, showers, information center

WHEELCHAIR ACCESS: No

COMMENTS: This trail begins at Algonquin Peak (page 296), and mileage begins at 4 miles.

CONTACTS: High Peaks trail information: www.dec.ny.gov/outdoor/9198.html; emergency contact: 518-891-0235

Overview

The initial descent from Algonquin Peak is bone jarring and punishing, 2,000 feet over 1.5 miles. Calling it a trail is a bit misleading; it's actually more like (and at times literally is) an active streambed. The good news is that the remainder of the trail, though rugged, is fairly level. The trail really stands out when you reach Avalanche Lake and head deeper into the pass. Steep cliffs and exposed mountain slides surround you as you hike literally suspended several feet above the lake. Combined with Algonquin Peak's stunning views and unique alpine zone, this trail is an amazing wilderness adventure but is recommended only for experienced hikers. Trail mileage begins with the 4-mile trek to reach Algonquin Peak.

Route Details

From Algonquin Peak, look for the rock cairns that head down along the southern slope of the mountain. Just as when you climbed to the summit, be careful to descend only along the trail/bedrock using rock cairns and pebble walls to help you navigate. A little over 0.3 mile and 400 feet along the descent, reach a fork in the trail that is encircled by shrub-sized evergreens. To the right/straight is the unmarked path to Boundary and Iroquois Peaks, while to the left is the main trail, indicated by an arrow and yellow trail markers. Just after this intersection, reach a steep drop and the alpine zone sign on this side of the mountain. The trail is now very narrow and is closed in by thick, shrub-sized spruces that gradually give way to taller trees as you quickly descend along the steep trail.

At 4.75 miles reach a steep descent that leads to a stream that tumbles through a cleft in the rock. This stream accompanies you—in fact much of the way it is the trail—as you descend the remaining 1,100 feet toward Lake Colden. Shortly after intersecting the stream, the trail heads away briefly only to wind back to the stream and, after descending a dilapidated log ladder, intersect it again at a tiny waterfall with a shallow pool at its base. From here forward, the trail

Avalanche Pass

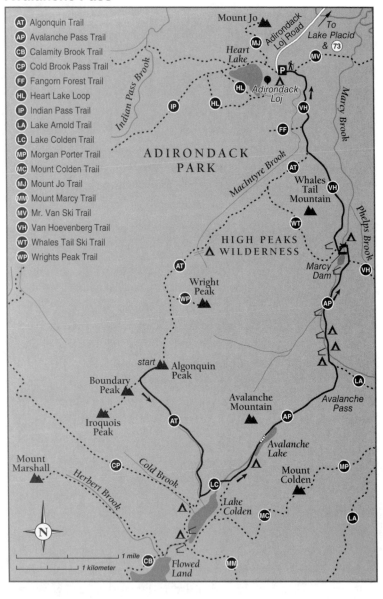

AT Algonquin Trail
AP Avalanche Pass Trail
CB Calamity Brook Trail
CP Cold Brook Pass Trail
FF Fangorn Forest Trail
HL Heart Lake Loop
IP Indian Pass Trail
LA Lake Arnold Trail
LC Lake Colden Trail
MP Morgan Porter Trail
MC Mount Colden Trail
MJ Mount Jo Trail
MM Mount Marcy Trail
MV Mr. Van Ski Trail
VH Van Hoevenberg Trail
WT Whales Tail Ski Trail
WP Wrights Peak Trail

Mount Jo
Adirondack Loj Road
To Lake Placid & 73

Heart Lake
MJ
MV

P
Adirondack Loj
HL
VH

Indian Pass Brook
IP
HL
FF

Marcy Brook

ADIRONDACK PARK

MacIntyre Brook
AT
Whales Tail Mountain
VH

Phelps Brook

WT

HIGH PEAKS
WILDERNESS

Marcy Dam
VH

AT
Wright Peak
WP
AP

LA

start Algonquin Peak
Boundary Peak
Avalanche Mountain
Avalanche Pass
AP

Iroquois Peak
AT

Mount Marshall
CP
Cold Brook
Herbert Brook
LC

Avalanche Lake

Mount Colden
MP

MC

Lake Colden
LA

N

1 mile
1 kilometer
CB
Flowed Land
MM

weaves back and forth and through the streambed, and finding the exact path while navigating the boulders and logs is tricky. To complicate things, there are a couple of trail reroutes along the descent, indicated by logs, branches, and rocks laid across the old trails. When in doubt, look for the yellow trail markers on the trees, and above all, be careful with your footing. Believe me, it is worth it.

When I made the descent, my foot slipped and my leg got caught between two rocks, deeply cutting my shin. It looked worse than it was, but it required eight stitches when I finally hobbled out hours later. I did not see anyone until I reached the final trail segment near the Loj parking area. Had my leg not popped out when trapped between the two rocks, it could have easily broken, turning a painful inconvenience into an outright disaster. It was a stark reminder that when in the wilderness, you are on your own and often self-rescue is your only option. Also, you are only as prepared as what you bring with you; a first aid kit (see page 17 for recommended items), extra food, flashlight or headlamp, and warm clothes are essential in the event you are forced to spend a night in the woods.

At 1.3 miles along the descent, the trail and stream follow a broad and open ledge a short way before reentering the forest on

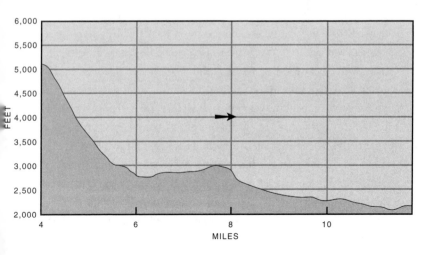

the north side of the stream. About 0.5 mile past this open ledge, the trail passes a tall waterfall with a shallow pool on the right. This waterfall roughly marks the end of the descent, and you soon reach a major trail intersection at 6 miles. To the right and over a log bridge, marked in yellow, is the trail to Lake Colden Dam/Outpost, as well as Cold Brook and Indian Pass Trails. Straight and marked in blue is the return leg of the loop to the Adirondack Loj via Avalanche Lake and Pass. Continue north through a marsh with several log-and-plank boardwalks and stunning views of the exposed slide on Mount Colden to the east. A third of a mile farther, 6.4 miles overall, reach another trail intersection and a trail register. To the right is Mount Colden via the northeast Mount Colden Trail, marked in yellow. Straight is the return to the Loj, now marked in yellow.

Continue north toward Avalanche Lake and Pass. Along this section of the trail, the stream between Avalanche Lake and Lake Colden flows on the left, and you will have to navigate a few mucky areas along the 0.3-mile stretch to Avalanche Lake. About midway, pass a camping disk, and the gap between Mount Colden to the east and Avalanche Mountain to the west visibly narrows. When you reach the tip of Avalanche Lake, you see that it is just a sliver of dark water between two sheer cliffs. The trail follows the west edge of the lake, and as the sheer cliff and lakeshore draw ever closer, you may begin to wonder where there is room for a trail. A quarter mile farther, you see that the answer is nowhere. The trail, an elevated boardwalk, has been literally attached to the sheer rock cliff and is suspended half a dozen feet above the dark lake. The boards are in pretty good shape, but wear and tear and seasonal damage make it prudent to test your footing and not put all your weight on a single board. This is the first of two elevated walks, and in between is a maze of boulders that you have to weave through and climb over. Log bridges and ladders assist in some of this trek, but be mindful of the condition of such aids as they are in a constant cycle of deterioration and replacement. It's a stunning scene, with evidence of recent slides (avalanches) throughout.

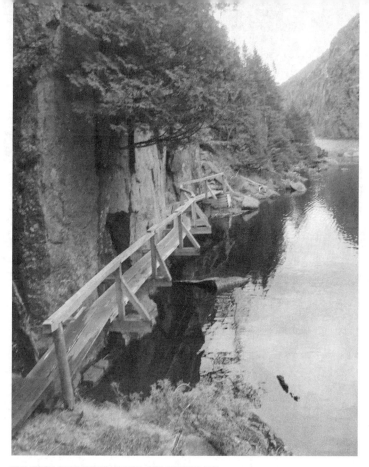

WALKWAY SUSPENDED ABOVE AVALANCHE LAKE

At 7.25 miles, the maze of boulders ends at the northern tip of Avalanche Lake. The trail continues north, heading deeper into the pass, first through a short muddy slog beside and through Avalanche Lake's feeder stream. Next is a narrow passage beside a steep cliff to the west, just before you reach the active avalanche area as indicated by the warning signs, 7.65 miles. Utterly clear of standing trees, the pass has an oddly unsteady feel underfoot because of the layers of mud and buried trees. After traversing to the western edge of the trail, you see how deep this fill is and why the ground has such a hollow feel. Slightly farther, you reach the end of the designated avalanche area, and the gradual descent to the Loj begins.

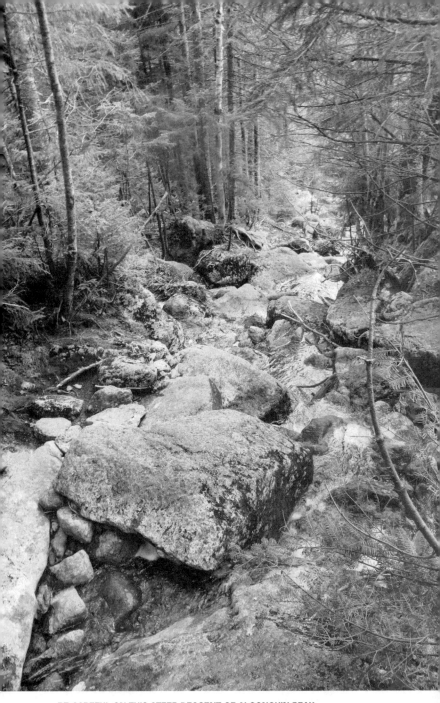

BE CAREFUL ON THIS STEEP DESCENT OF ALGONQUIN PEAK.

At 8.4 miles reach the intersection with the Lake Arnold Trail, marked in blue on the right. Continue straight toward the Adirondack Loj, still marked in yellow. Shortly after the intersection, reach a bridge with handrails that crosses Marcy Brook; this brook will accompany you the whole way north to the interior campsites and lean-tos near Marcy Dam, a little more than 0.75 mile ahead. You will pass a couple of lean-tos along this trek, along with several designated camping areas, before you reach the intersection with the Van Hoevenberg Trail, on the right and marked in blue, 9.4 miles overall. Bear left and continue north past the trail register a short ways to another intersection, this time indicating the direction to the Adirondack Loj and path forward. Continue left past the remains of Marcy Dam toward the Loj, now following blue disks for the rest of the trail, and soon reach a bridge that crosses Marcy Brook a few hundred feet north of the dam. Once across, the trail swings briefly south to intersect where it used to cross Marcy Dam and then continues its northerly descent. The remaining 2.2 miles back to the Loj follow a highly traveled and well-maintained section. At 10.8 miles reintersect the trail to Algonquin with only 1 mile remaining back along the original route to the Loj and parking area for a total loop of 11.8 miles.

Directions

From the intersection of NY 73 and NY 86 in Lake Placid, head 3.3 miles south on NY 73, and follow the directions below. From the intersection of NY 73 and NY 9N in downtown Keene, head 10.9 miles west on NY 73, and follow the directions below.

Turn south onto Adirondack Loj Road. Continue 5.1 miles to the vehicle-entry booth, and the main parking area is on the left past the visitor center.

44 Little and Big Crow Mountains

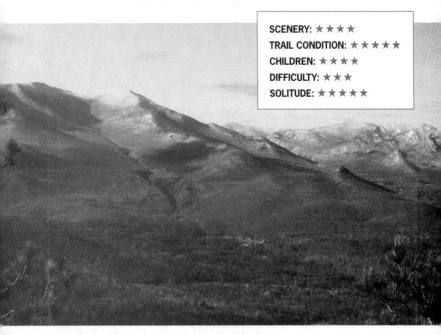

SCENERY: ★ ★ ★ ★
TRAIL CONDITION: ★ ★ ★ ★ ★
CHILDREN: ★ ★ ★ ★
DIFFICULTY: ★ ★ ★
SOLITUDE: ★ ★ ★ ★ ★

LOOKING OUT ON THE HIGH PEAKS FROM BIG CROW

GPS COORDINATES: N44° 15.696'   W73° 44.010'

DISTANCE & CONFIGURATION: 3.3-mile loop

HIKING TIME: 2–3 hours

HIGHLIGHTS: Spectacular vistas

ELEVATION: 1,742' at trailhead, 2,800' at highest point

ACCESS: Open 24/7; no fees or permits required

MAPS: Hurricane Mountain Wilderness map: tinyurl.com/hurricanemtnmap; National Geographic *Adirondack Park, Lake Placid/High Peaks* (#742)

FACILITIES: None

WHEELCHAIR ACCESS: No

CONTACTS: High Peaks Adirondack trail information: www.dec.ny.gov/outdoor/9198.html; Hurricane Mountain Wilderness: www.dec.ny.gov/lands/100895.html; emergency contact: 518-891-0235

Overview

This short trip is an excellent introductory hike for those who want to familiarize themselves with the beautiful vistas of the High Peaks without spending a whole day. Both experts and novices will appreciate the wealth of views atop the many ledges you encounter as you weave your way to the summit.

Route Details

To make the trail into a loop, you will have to walk 1.4 miles along O'Toole Road and Hurricane Road. You can hike the road section either at the end or at the beginning of the hike, but I recommend hiking the trail clockwise and including the roadside portion at the beginning. The counterclockwise direction includes a steeper ascent to Big Crow and requires you to end your hike walking uphill along the road rather than with a descent and flat stroll through the woods.

The trail register is located a few hundred yards northwest of the parking area. To reach the western trailhead, walk down O'Toole Road, and turn right onto Hurricane Road, 1.1 miles. Continue down Hurricane Road 0.2 mile, and look for a small orange ADK marker affixed to a wooden sign that points to the trail. This sign is difficult to see while driving but evident while on foot. The trail starts at a couple of log steps and winds around the left side of a private residence. This section of the trail is on private property, so be careful to stay on the marked portion of the trail.

Red trail disks mark the way, and you quickly begin to climb through a stand of small saplings. Roughly 0.5 mile into the trail, 1.8 miles from the start, expansive views to the south and west begin to open up behind you. Exposed portions of bedrock begin to jut out, both making the terrain more rugged and forming natural steps as you climb. You will see yellow paint blazes on trees that may seem to guide you along the trail, but these are actually the boundary between private property and the Hurricane Mountain Wilderness.

Little and Big Crow Mountains

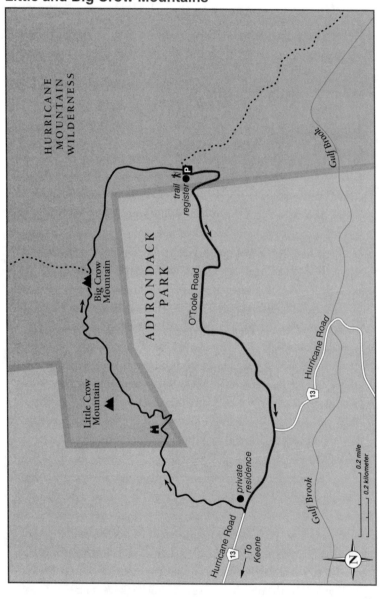

The exposed ledges along the trail all offer wonderful views, but a particularly spectacular vista is available just past where you enter the public lands, 2 miles from the start. Take advantage of these lookouts, as the summit of Little Crow does not offer any views. Red disks and rock cairns help you navigate as you weave your way over exposed portions of bedrock and through windswept conifers. At 2.3 miles the peak of Little Crow Mountain (2,450') is off to the left of the main trail. The bald top of Little Crow is quite exposed, but it is also a broad peak; consequently, the encircling evergreens limit views typical of a bald summit.

To reach Big Crow, continue east along the exposed bedrock, and then quickly descend the short pass between the two peaks. Big Crow appears more rugged as you approach, but the climb to Little Crow is actually the tougher of the two. The oak saplings that fill the pass are a pleasant diversion from the encompassing evergreens that shroud the mountaintops. Indeed, as you climb Big Crow, the conifers become dense, and they so closely flank the trail that only the path ahead is visible. However, the dense foliage is brief, and a view north soon rewards your efforts. Whiteface Mountain, with its numerous ski slopes, is particularly prominent as you look north.

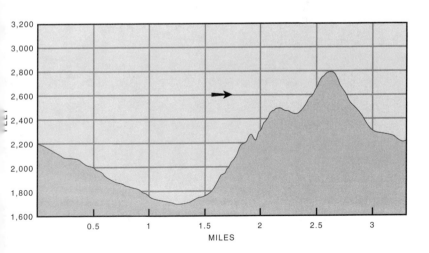

The trail turns south, and a lookout south and west quickly reveals the path you have taken. After a brief scramble up the exposed bedrock, you reach the beginning of the exposed spine that runs along the short ridge. A sweeping panorama of tall peaks extends from due east southward to due west as you traverse the ridge. The highest point on the trip (2,800') is at 2.8 miles and is simply atop a boulder where a sign reminds visitors that no camping or fires are allowed at the peak. Continue east along the ridge to where the descent of the open face is rather steep. After approximately 0.25 mile the steep section is past, and the rest of the hike through the spruce forest feels very sheltered compared with the exposed peaks. At 3.2 miles you cross a small brook, after which the trail is mostly level, and you quickly reach the trail register and return to the parking area approximately 0.25 mile ahead.

Directions

From the intersection of NY 9N and NY 73 in downtown Keene, head southeast on NY 73/NY 9N, and turn left onto County Road 13/Hurricane Road (1.7 miles north of the southern intersection of NY 73 and NY 9N, and 0.2 mile south of the northern intersection of NY 73 and NY 9N). Continue on CR 13/Hurricane Road 2.3 miles, and turn left onto O'Toole Road. Follow O'Toole Road 1.1 miles to the parking area at the end.

Pitchoff Mountain

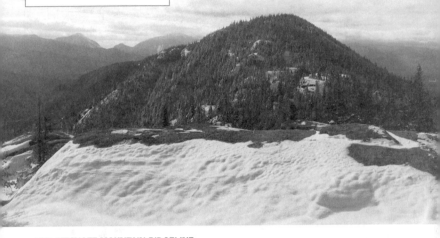

SCENERY: ★ ★ ★ ★ ★
TRAIL CONDITION: ★ ★ ★ ★
CHILDREN: ★ ★ ★
DIFFICULTY: ★ ★ ★ ★
SOLITUDE: ★ ★ ★ ★

THE PITCHOFF MOUNTAIN RIDGELINE

GPS COORDINATES: East trailhead: N44° 14.624'   W73° 50.752'
West trailhead: N44° 13.172'   W73° 53.175'

DISTANCE & CONFIGURATION: 4.6-mile point-to-point

HIKING TIME: 5–6 hours

HIGHLIGHTS: Panoramic views, open ledges

ELEVATION: 1,850' at trailhead, 3,600' at highest point along the trail

ACCESS: Open 24/7; no fees or permits required

MAPS: Sentinel Range Wilderness map: tinyurl.com/sentinelrangemap; National Geographic *Adirondack Park, Lake Placid/High Peaks* (#742)

FACILITIES: None

WHEELCHAIR ACCESS: No

CONTACTS: High Peaks Adirondack trail information: www.dec.ny.gov/outdoor/9198.html; Sentinel Range Wilderness: www.dec.ny.gov/lands/101901.html; emergency contact: 518-891-0235

Pitchoff Mountain

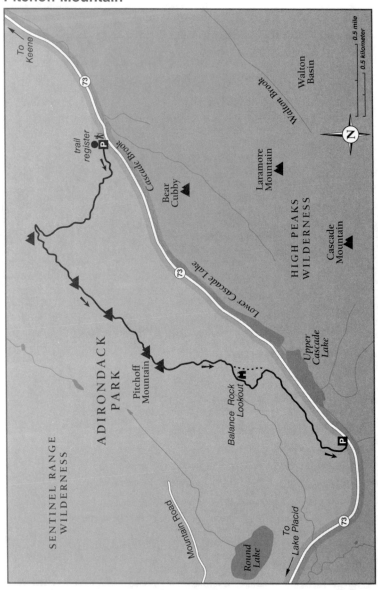

Overview

This rocky ridge parallels NY 73 and provides wonderful views of the High Peaks wilderness to the south. This is an end-to-end hike and easiest to manage with two cars—or park at one end and catch a ride to the other. There are several steep rock scrambles, so be prepared during wet and icy conditions.

Route Details

The two trailheads are 2.7 miles apart along NY 73. This is a major road with narrow shoulders, so it is advised that you either leave a vehicle at both ends or leave your car at one end and get a lift to the other. I would suggest getting a ride before your hike, rather than after, to avoid uncertainty and because the trail will likely take longer than is typical for the mileage. The west trailhead has more parking room, so it is best to leave your vehicle there and hike the trail from east to west. Directions below are given in that direction.

The east trailhead is little more than a worn path with a couple of steps that extend down to the road, but there are signs, and it is distinct. The trail register is at the beginning of the trail, and

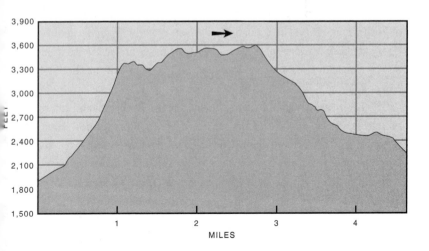

even though you will sign in and out at different registers, it is still important to sign in and out. The trail, marked with red disks and yellow blazes for the whole trip, turns west almost immediately and parallels the road roughly 0.3 mile under a canopy of birch and beech trees. The trail swings north, and you begin climbing among a jumble of cobbles and boulders alongside a rocky brook. The grade steadily increases and becomes a lot steeper 0.8 mile into the hike. At approximately 1 mile you have almost reached the ridge that you will traverse, and though many steep up-and-down sections are still ahead, the majority of the climbing is behind you. At 1.1 miles you pass through a wet area between two 20- to 30-foot-high rocky outcrops that flank the trail. After this small pass, the trail turns left, and you scramble up to the top of one of these outcrops.

At 1.2 miles you have reached the first of five minor peaks that make up Pitchoff Mountain. Ridgelines with multiple peaks do not have separate mountain names if the prominence of a peak does not exceed 980 feet or 7–8% relative prominence above the highest saddle or col between the peaks. In ridges such as this one, with slight elevation differences between peaks and cols, it's clear why the distinction between mountains and peaks is useful. The trail weaves its way up and down many times before you reach the actual summit, 1.5 miles ahead. The views south are exceptional, and many similar vantage points will accompany you as you traverse the spine. Yellow paint blazes mark the path along these bald peaks. If you are attempting this hike after a recent snowfall, finding your way can be time consuming. Snow falls as early as October and as late as spring in the High Peaks region. During the light snows of the fall and thaws during spring, when the snow is not deep enough for snowshoes, you need crampons or their equivalent to cross the bald peaks. The cycles of thawing and freezing on the exposed rocky ledges and peaks produce sheets of ice that are treacherous without added traction. Pack accordingly, even though these conditions may not be evident down at the road.

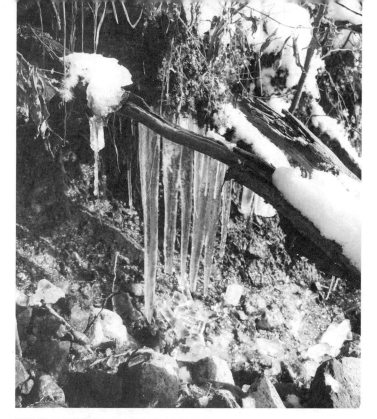

ICICLES ALONG THE TRAIL IN EARLY OCTOBER

The trail weaves up and down over boulders and zigzags through wind-stunted evergreens across the entire spine. Many times you will think that you have reached a peak or traversed a pass between peaks, only to find yet another climb or pass before you. This is particularly true for the 0.5 mile between the first and second peaks. The second peak, 1.8 miles overall, offers a wide panoramic view south but does not offer the 360-degree views found at the first peak. The trail descends and climbs mostly along the ridgeline to the third peak at 2.1 miles, where there are also views south.

Between the third and fourth summits, the trail meanders to the north side of the ridge, where the fir trees become thick, and then heads back to the south side. The fourth peak, 2.5 miles, is not the highest point of elevation but is the last peak with panoramic views.

At 2.7 miles you pass some balancing boulders that mark the fifth and final peak as well as the beginning of the steep descent from the ridgeline. Dense conifers shroud the trail for most of the descent, but occasional breaks in the trails and open ledges offer some views.

At 3.2 miles you reach the only fork in the trail and a sign that indicates a view is off to the left. This lookout, approximately 0.1 mile along an unmarked path, is atop a sheer ledge with two balanced boulders that sit at its westernmost edge. Cascade Mountain and Upper and Lower Cascade Lakes are the prominent features of the view, and the lookout is certainly worth the short side trip.

Back along the trail, the descent is much steeper, and the forest transitions back to hardwoods. The steep descent continues about 0.5 mile, during which you pass under the sheer rock wall that makes up the lookout to your left. The trail turns west, levels off, and parallels NY 73 and Upper Cascade Lake for the next 0.5 mile. At 4.3 miles, the trail swings south, and you descend for the next 0.3 mile until you reach the western trailhead and Upper Cascade Lake parking area.

Directions

Parking is available at both the east and west ends of Cascade Lake along NY 73. Parking is limited in both areas, and there is little room on the roadside. The parking areas are 2.7 miles apart along NY 73.

From the northern intersection of NY 73 and NY 9N in downtown Keene, head 3.9 miles west on NY 73 to the east parking area. Head 6.6 miles west on NY 73 to reach the west parking area.

From the intersection of County Road 21 and NY 73, near the Olympic ski jump in Lake Placid, head 5.6 miles east to the west parking area or 8.3 miles east to the east parking area.

Ampersand Mountain

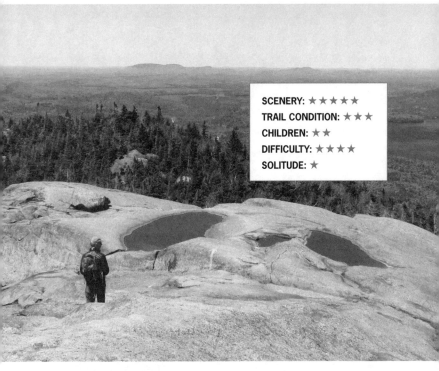

SCENERY: ★ ★ ★ ★ ★
TRAIL CONDITION: ★ ★ ★
CHILDREN: ★ ★
DIFFICULTY: ★ ★ ★ ★
SOLITUDE: ★

ON TOP OF AMPERSAND MOUNTAIN

GPS COORDINATES: N44° 15.095'   W74° 14.374'

DISTANCE & CONFIGURATION: 5.2-mile out-and-back

HIKING TIME: 3–4 hours

HIGHLIGHTS: Bald summit, panoramic views

ELEVATION: 1,550' at trailhead, 3,353' at highest point

ACCESS: Open 24/7; no fees or permits required

MAPS: National Geographic *Adirondack Park, Lake Placid/High Peaks* (#742)

FACILITIES: None

WHEELCHAIR ACCESS: No

CONTACTS: High Peaks Adirondack trail information: www.dec.ny.gov/outdoor/9198.html;
emergency contact: 518-891-0235

Ampersand Mountain

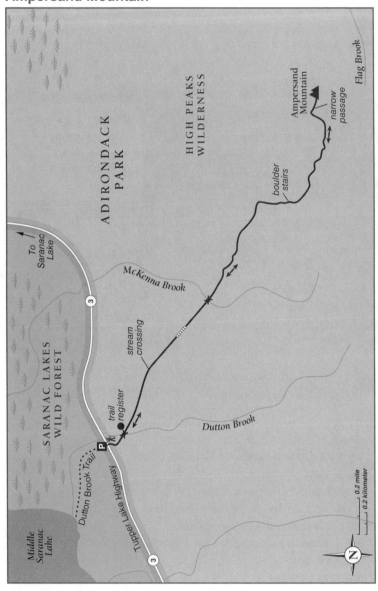

Overview

Ampersand Mountain sits on the confluence of the flat north and High Peaks regions of the Adirondacks. An extremely popular hike, it offers a varied experience as you transition from a gentle walk through tall hemlocks to a steep ascent over boulder stairs. Passage through enormous, craggy boulders takes you to the bald summit, from which the lake sprawls out beneath you to the north and the High Peaks can be seen in the distance to the south.

Route Details

When I approached on a sunny Saturday afternoon, it was clear that this trail is extremely popular. Dozens of cars lined NY 3 on both sides, and I could see that the small parking area was nowhere near adequate. While the lot also provides access to a short trail to Dutton Brook, the vast majority of hikers were climbing Ampersand Mountain. Indeed the trail register had been filled days before by the dozens of parties that hike the trail each day during the peak of summer. As with all popular trails, it is best to visit these in the off-season, during the week, or early if you have any desire for privacy.

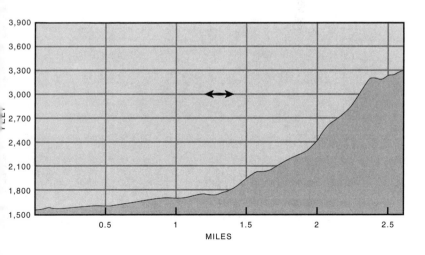

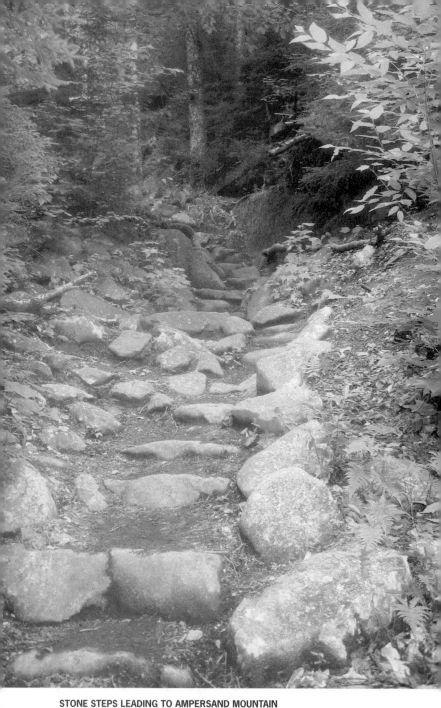

STONE STEPS LEADING TO AMPERSAND MOUNTAIN

Why is the trail so popular? It is likely that the combination of the easy stroll at the beginning through towering old-growth forest, its proximity to a major road and tourist destinations, and the spectacular views all contribute to its appeal. Unfortunately, I reached the summit when a major thunderstorm had rolled in and visibility had dropped to several feet, so I cannot attest to the latter. The peak was awash in a sheet of flowing rain, and I was stuck in a cloud. Lightning flashed in all directions, and fierce winds threatened to blow others and me off the peak. Lingering in these conditions was unwise at best, so I did not get to see the views that people raved about, but according to veterans of this hike, the views are breathtaking and panoramic. It was a stark reminder that even though it is sunny and clear at the start of a hike, conditions can change quickly, and a little precaution and preparation are required on every hike and in every season.

Update: Having revisited the trail, I can attest that the views atop Ampersand are spectacular. When I originally visited, visibility was limited to a few feet, so I was surprised on returning to find how broad and spread out the peak is. Even on a crowded Saturday/holiday weekend, there was space for numerous groups to find spots to sit and enjoy the views while resting before their descent. There are several spots with 360-degree views, but on windy days it is likely you will want to shelter in one of the many dips/crevices, of which there are several.

The trailhead is on the southern side of NY 3 across from the small parking area. The trail register is just inside the woods, and the wide and gravelly base attests to the heavy use and ongoing maintenance. In less than 0.3 mile, you cross Dutton Brook over a log bridge. Shortly after this crossing, you will definitely notice the towering hemlocks, which are some of the few remaining old-growth trees in the Adirondacks. This forest is considered the largest known sugar maple–yellow birch–hemlock forest in Adirondack Park. Red disks mark the trail, but it is so heavily trodden that, except for a few places near the summit where blowdown occurs, they are hardly necessary. At 0.8 mile, planks laid lengthwise form a boardwalk over a wet area. At 1 mile, you cross McKenna Brook over a log bridge.

Past this crossing, the trail begins to climb, and you will rock-hop across streams and more mucky areas as the trail gradually becomes steep. The hemlocks that previously towered overhead give way to birches and maples, and the vast stonework employed to control erosion becomes evident. Long stretches of boulder stairs were constructed within the past decade to minimize the impact hikers had on the trail, once considered one of the most heavily eroded. Climbing only on the stone sections gives the forest a chance to regenerate some of its ground cover and, hopefully, forestalls further erosion. The last mile is basically a vertical climb, and you may need to use your hands.

As the forest transitions from hardwoods to stunted firs and evergreens, the stonework diminishes until it becomes nonexistent, and the erosion becomes severe. At this point, the various paths chosen to bypass washed-out areas or precipitous sections make finding the trail difficult and trail markers a necessity. Take your time throughout the final climb, and use caution over eroded and slippery surfaces.

Around 2.3 miles, the trail levels off briefly just shy of the summit. You pass a few large boulders and eventually come to a passage between exposed faces of bedrock with a fissure opening up on your right. The trail then turns left and winds around to a rock face that you must scramble up and over. The roots of a tree will help you up, but after seeing the erosion caused by so many hikers, you can't help but wonder how much longer this tree will be around. Yellow arrows painted on the bald mountaintop point you in the direction of the easiest ways around the three knobs. Many of the bald peaks in the Adirondacks were created when Verplanck Colvin burned the tops of mountains during his 19th-century survey of the region. Erosion soon swept away the topsoil, leaving the mountains bald. Each knob offers its own merits and vantage points, and curious hikers will also find the remnants of a fire tower, as well as

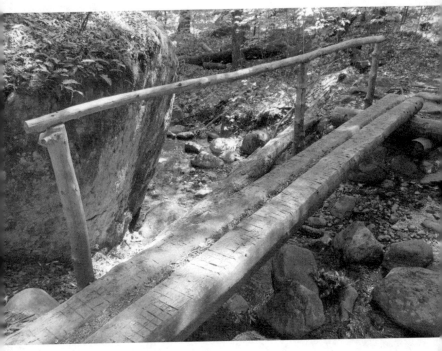

LOG BRIDGE ALONG THE TRAIL

a plaque in memory of the Ampersand Hermit. The hermit, Walter Channing Rice, manned the fire tower from 1915 to 1923.

Directions

FROM THE WEST　From Tupper Lake, head east on NY 3/NY 30. At 5.3 miles, bear right to stay on NY 3. After another 6.9 miles, the designated parking area is on your left. The parking area may be full, so take care when parking on the side of the road.

FROM THE EAST　From the intersection of NY 3 and NY 86 in Saranac Lake, head 8.4 miles west on NY 3; the parking area is on the right.

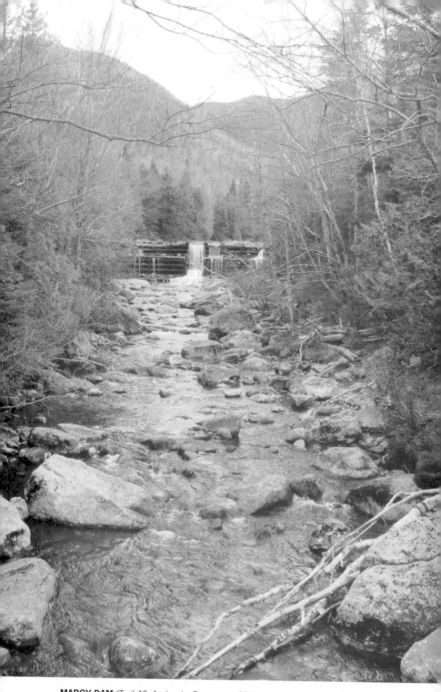

MARCY DAM (Trail 43, Avalanche Pass, page 304)

Appendix A: Managing Agencies

ADIRONDACK PARK AGENCY

apa.state.ny.us

518-891-4050

NEW YORK STATE DEPARTMENT OF ENVIRONMENTAL CONSERVATION

www.dec.ny.gov

Region 5 (Eastern Adirondacks): Essex, Hamilton, Warren, Fulton, Saratoga, and Washington Counties: 518-897-1200

Region 6 (Western Adirondacks): Jefferson, St. Lawrence, Lewis, Oneida, and Herkimer Counties: 518-785-2239

Forest Ranger Emergency Contact: 518-891-0235

Appendix B: Gear Lists

Day Hike Gear List

THE ESSENTIALS

Backpack

Boots

Extra food

First aid kit

Flashlight and extra batteries

Pocketknife or multitool

This book

Topographical map and compass

Water bottles

Water filter or purification tablets

Waterproof matches and/or lighter, as well as a fire starter

Whistle

ADDITIONAL

Change of clothes

Extra socks

Insect repellent

Personal medications

Poncho or raingear

UV sunblock and lip balm

Warm hat

OPTIONAL

Camera with extra batteries and memory cards

Gaiters

Garbage bag for packing out trash

GPS unit

Repair kit

Small towel

Swimsuit

Survival kit

Toilet paper

Trowel or small shovel for digging catholes

Summer Backpacking Gear List

Backpack

Bear bag or canister

Cleaning supplies (biodegradable detergent and container, sponge, and scouring pad)

Collapsible bucket or water bag

Collapsible pillow

Cooking pots and pans

Eating utensils (cup, bowl, plate, knife, fork, and spoon)

Food (including extra for emergencies)

Garbage bag for packing out trash

Rope and nylon cord (50 feet)

Shelter and conveyance

Sleeping bag and sleeping pad or mattress

Stove and fuel

Tent and rain fly

Tent stakes

Water bottles

Water filter or purification tablets

Waterproof matches and/or lighter, as well as a fire starter

PERSONAL ITEMS

Biodegradable hand soap

First aid kit

Insect repellent

Personal medications

Small towel

Toilet paper

Toothbrush and toothpaste

Trowel or small shovel for digging catholes

UV sunblock and lip balm

GEAR

Camera with extra batteries and memory cards

Camp light or candle

Flashlight and extra batteries

GPS unit

Pocketknife or multitool

Repair kit

Sewing kit

Stuff sacks

Survival kit

This book

Topographical map and compass

Whistle

CLOTHING

Boots

Camp shoes

Extra socks

Gaiters

Jacket or outerwear (layer clothing)

Light shirt or T-shirt

Long pants

Plastic bag for laundry

Poncho or raingear

Shorts

Sock liners

Swimsuit

Warm hat

Warm shirt

Appendix C: Hiking Clubs

ADIRONDACK MOUNTAIN CLUB
Includes many local chapters in New York and beyond
adk.org

ADK46ERS
Nonprofit that focuses on the ultimate Adirondack bucket list
adk46er.org

Appendix D: Suggested Reading

Dunn, Russell. *Adirondack Waterfall Guide: New York's Cool Cascades.* Delmar, NY: Black Dome Press Corp., 2004. Out of print.

Ketchledge, Edwin H. *Forests and Trees of the Adirondack High Peaks Region: A Hiker's Guide.* Lake George, NY: Adirondack Mountain Club, 1996.

Starmer, Tim. *Five-Star Trails: Finger Lakes & Central New York.* Birmingham, AL: Menasha Ridge Press, 2014.

Van Diver, Bradford B. *Roadside Geology of New York.* Missoula, MT: Mountain Press Publishing Company, 1985.

Starmer, Aaron, and Cate Starmer and Tim Starmer. *Best Tent Camping: New York State.* Birmingham, AL: Menasha Ridge Press, 2013.

Index

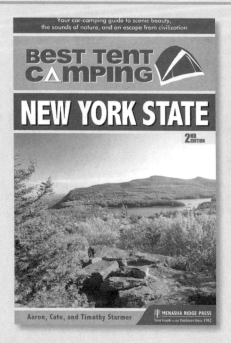

About the Author

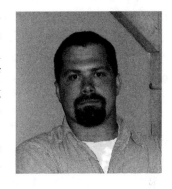

TIM STARMER has always been an out-doors enthusiast and spent most of his childhood seeking out remote and wild areas whenever possible. During a brief hiatus from Brown University during 1997, he drove across the United States for six weeks, camping the entire way. Along the way he explored many of the West's national and state parks, including Canyonlands, Yellowstone, Arches, and Bryce Canyon—he even braved pitching a tent among the mosquito swarms in Badlands National Park. At the trip's conclusion, he headed down to Australia, where he backpacked for a few months exploring the eastern outback, the Great Barrier Reef, and the caves of Tasmania, as well as traversing the Tasmanian Wilderness World Heritage Area along the Overland Track. Starmer owns and operates New Heritage Woodworking, a construction company that specializes in designing and building timber frames, and he can still be found exploring the wilds whenever possible.

DEAR CUSTOMERS AND FRIENDS,

SUPPORTING YOUR INTEREST IN OUTDOOR ADVENTURE, travel, and an active lifestyle is central to our operations, from the authors we choose to the locations we detail to the way we design our books. Menasha Ridge Press was incorporated in 1982 by a group of veteran outdoorsmen and professional outfitters. For many years now, we've specialized in creating books that benefit the outdoors enthusiast.

Almost immediately, Menasha Ridge Press earned a reputation for revolutionizing outdoors- and travel-guidebook publishing. For such activities as canoeing, kayaking, hiking, backpacking, and mountain biking, we established new standards of quality that transformed the whole genre, resulting in outdoor-recreation guides of great sophistication and solid content. Menasha Ridge Press continues to be outdoor publishing's greatest innovator.

The folks at Menasha Ridge Press are as at home on a whitewater river or mountain trail as they are editing a manuscript. The books we build for you are the best they can be, because we're responding to your needs. Plus, we use and depend on them ourselves.

We look forward to seeing you on the river or the trail. If you'd like to contact us directly, visit us at menasharidge.com. We thank you for your interest in our books and the natural world around us all.

SAFE TRAVELS,

BOB SEHLINGER
PUBLISHER